Plants R Cures

An Almanac of Plants & Medicine

Martin E. Gordon, M.D.

Copyright © 2019 Martin E. Gordon, M.D.

All rights reserved. No part of this book may be used or reproduced by any means, graphic, electronic, or mechanical, including photocopying, recording, taping or by any information storage retrieval system without the written permission of the author except in the case of brief quotations embodied in critical articles and reviews.

The information, ideas, and suggestions in this book are not intended as a substitute for professional medical advice. Before following any suggestions contained in this book, you should consult your personal physician. Neither the author nor the publisher shall be liable or responsible for any loss or damage allegedly arising as a consequence of your use or application of any information or suggestions in this book.

LifeRich Publishing is a registered trademark of The Reader's Digest Association, Inc.

LifeRich Publishing books may be ordered through booksellers or by contacting:

LifeRich Publishing
1663 Liberty Drive
Bloomington, IN 47403
www.liferichpublishing.com
1 (888) 238-8637

Because of the dynamic nature of the Internet, any web addresses or links contained in this book may have changed since publication and may no longer be valid. The views expressed in this work are solely those of the author and do not necessarily reflect the views of the publisher, and the publisher hereby disclaims any responsibility for them.

Any people depicted in stock imagery provided by Getty Images are models, and such images are being used for illustrative purposes only.
Certain stock imagery © Getty Images.

ISBN: 978-1-4897-2205-8 (sc)
ISBN: 978-1-4897-2206-5 (e)

Library of Congress Control Number: 2019940436

Print information available on the last page.

LifeRich Publishing rev. date: 5/8/2019

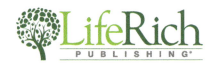

Would you like to watch some of the leading experts on plants and biomedicine discuss their work? The *Plants R Cures* **YouTube channel** features the author's interviews with outstanding plant science researchers.

Go to www.youtube.com/channel/UCLx_CyIkm5p6PfZsT_OlOhw.

Dedicated to

Evelyn E. Gordon and Madelon T. Price

Who inspired this work

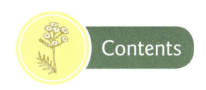

Contents

- Beginnings 1
- How Intelligent Is Your Ficus? 4
- A Few Basic Benefits to Start With 5
- Plant Science Origins 6
- …Vs Our Modern Diet (how different are we?) 6
- Plant Pigments, pt 1 — what do they tell us? 7
- Mushrooms R Medicine — the good news 8
- The Good & the Bad 10
- What Your Ancestors Knew 14
- The Lessons of Patient Histories (be patient) 14
- Hooked on Hooke — & other pioneers & key inventions 18
- Peter Raven — a note of wisdom 27
- Plant Pigments, pt 2 27
- Photosynthesis — plant energy 28
- Beer — as old as civilization 29
- Plant Scientists — the early explorers and innovators 31
- Crop Biotechnology Today (with a nod to Jefferson) 36
- Trees & Leaves & Us 38
- Pollinators & Colony Collapse 41
- Short Notes — stem cells, weeds, marijuana (*the* weed) & ginger 42
- On to Herbals 43
- What Are Your Symptoms? — consider plants (& pesticides) 44
- Getting Quizzical 45

- Correlation of Signs & Symptoms — a comprehensive Plants R Cures chart 46
- What About Tea? 55
- Medical Devices & Innovations — from obsidian scalpels to nanoparticles 56
- Parasitic Diseases & Neglected Tropical Diseases — do not neglect the plants 58
- Global Hazards for Expatriates — toxins, carcinogens and other potential treacheries 59
- Ruminations on Travel Medicine by an Armchair Clinician 64
- A Planter's Sampler Box for the Curious 65
- Glossary: In a Word 66
- In Closing 67
- Some Key Works 67
- Plant Libraries for Exploration 69
- Last Words — Acknowledgments 70

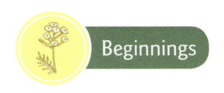

Beginnings

Nature was the first Nanotechnologist

We invariably recall repressed failures, interspersed occasionally with euphoric joy. Such was an event that occurred the summer in Ohio that I was Waterfront Director at a children's summer camp. My fluid swimming instructions were interrupted by the camp's loudspeaker shouting at me to "come to the dining room immediately!!" That single telegram from Yale University changed my life completely, as I had abruptly become the first Kent State University student offered admission to the Yale Medical School. Imagine experiencing the prior disconcerting 21 rejection letters from other medical institutions, followed by that incredible pronouncement of acceptance.

This eBook reflects my attempts during my subsequent journey to increase the awareness of the virtuous contributions of plants to improve the clinical care of patients. Hopefully, reading this eBook may become an informative as well as enjoyable experience.

> *All that man needs for health and healing has been provided by God in nature, the challenge of science is to find it.*
> ~ Paracelsus, Swiss philosopher, physician, botanist, 1493–1540

This panoramic eBook *Plants R Cures* strives to ignite and excite interest in our silent green plant alchemy and point out the ways that plants can ameliorate disease, feed the world and provide solutions to energy and industrial needs. Appropriate cautions about side effects and sustainability losses are presented for all healthcare workers, amalgamating health dysfunctions with solutions for treating global disease. The graphics with text lessons lead to better understanding of clinical symptoms, along with vividly illustrated case histories.

Beneficial evidenced-based plant products are itemized, e.g.: ginger for nausea associated with pregnancy or seasickness; curcumin (turmeric) for NASH and irritable bowel syndrome; milk thistle for hepatic dysfunction related to mushroom or acetaminophen poisoning; and Manuka honey for resistant MRSA and H. pylori infections.

Close to one third of modern prescription medicines contain a plant-derived ingredient, and chemicals from plants have contributed to the production of many synthetic compounds and pharmaceuticals (e.g. cashew nut liquid is added to paints utilized by the US navy to prevent rust and fires). Biosphere images are now used to detect plant pests' chemical signatures, leading to protein tools for reshaping genomes.

> *A diagnosis is easy, as long as you think of it*
> ~ Soma Weiss

The text includes a history of plant discovery, their many environmental and personal challenges, and the fearless explorers and purveyors of the plant trade. The *Plants Have Feelings Too* text explains how plants revise their molecular structure in response to environmental challenge; evidence-based herbal use; and cautionary tales of plant-related toxicity. It addresses plants as beauty aids and as sources of untapped nutrition and vitamins, as well as the use of nuisance species—weeds that may still fill our needs. Each topic includes possible future research.

This book is designed to be accessible to everyone—the patient seeking improved health and well-being, the concerned parent, health care workers, sleuthing clinicians, plant lovers and the curious. It is designed for bio-medical students, individuals interested in working in the field of plant science, and those who simply want to learn more about herbal remedies to treat current medical conditions and ailments and to begin making choices for a healthier life.

Today scientists are making awesome discoveries employing nanotechnology. Their work has led to understanding common daily fractals, which consist of common repeating patterns that are infinitely small and yet speed our understanding of nature's unrelenting botanical rhythmic patterns.

Seldom do we recall that tree branches, flower petals, snail contours, river flows, broccoli, heartbeat irregularities and our own lung bronchi are composed of duplicating patterns. These all express a seemingly chaotic image, yet we must invoke new thinking as

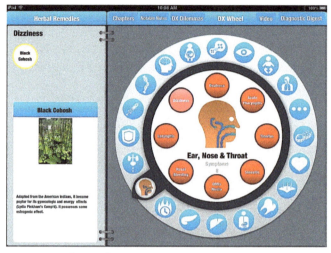

From author's Plants 4 Cures app (courtesy of author)

the technology unfolds, for a better understanding of Nature's unrelenting "chaotic," yet pseudo-orderly, patterns. This book will attempt to correlate the ongoing interaction of plants, animals and humans, hopefully harvesting health as we seek to understand how *Plants R Cures*.

Puzzled by fractals? Do not be hesitant to read on. The discoverer Benoit Mandelbrot's own definition is that "a fractal is a geometric shape that can be separated into parts, each of which is a reduced-scale version of the whole." Think nesting Russian Dolls repeating their own images. Read more at: https://phys.org/news/2011-02-experimental-scale.html.

We can now get a glimpse of the speed of biochemical reactions within plants, via compressed ultrafast photography, at 100 billion frames/second. With this knowledge we can continue to be humbled by the universe's vastness and also by the information available, using the newest

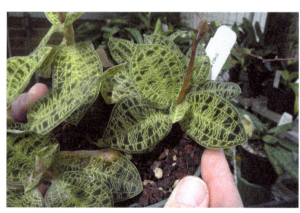

Fractals in leaves (courtesy of author)

technological techniques for deciphering plant genomes, which are bigger and more complex than the human genome. They too lead to a better understanding of the mysteries of nature.

Since opening my consulting practice of gastroenterology in 1954, I've welcomed the opportunity to share with patients, their families, and "younger neophytes" knowledge of the healing power of plants. My enthusiasm widens with time, never dimming or dulling as challenges are confronted daily. I marvel at the remarkable current imaging with endoscopic, genetic enhancers and other diagnostic devices, and at the many treatment aids now readily available.

Working as an active licensed physician, mentor and patient advocate, I continue to see patients at a free clinic in St Louis while engaging in plant-related projects. *Plants R Cures* is about finding healthier healing sources in plants, enhancing patient care and expanding the herbalist culture.

Additionally, I believe that Complementary Alternative Medicine (CAM), also now referred to as Integrated and Precision Medicine, has a place in medicine today. Choosing alternative treatment is becoming more acceptable: it is a trend I applaud and will discuss as we move forward together. Throughout this book, I'll draw on my decades-long career in medicine and offer you, the readers, a brief history of some little known but always fascinating "medical stories."

Trained medical doctors use every tool available to restore health and vitality. Patients should be equally passionate about their own health choices. Or as Immanuel Kant suggested: "Have the courage to use your own intelligence!"

The pseudo-separation of botany and medicine as disciplines may be compared to companions that occasionally separate but become symbiotic along the way. The partnership of plants and medicine is explained in this book.

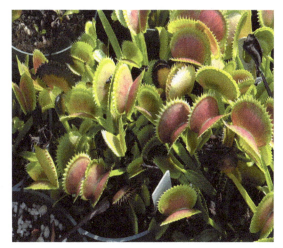

Carnivorous plants (courtesy of author)

Writing this book is my attempt to share fascinating knowledge, hoping your experience in reading it will lead you to a meaningful, long and healthy life.

How Intelligent Is Your Ficus?

Summary of Challenges

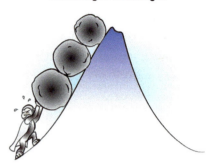

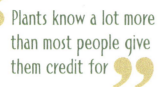

> "Plants know a lot more than most people give them credit for"
> ~ The American Gardener

> "How does a Venus flytrap know when to snap shut? Can an orchid get jet lag? Does a tomato plant feel pain when you pluck a fruit from its vines? And does your favorite fern care whether you play Bach or the Beatles?"
> ~ Daniel Chamovitz

That plants have a far greater ability to sense their world than appearances might suggest has led to some remarkable claims about "plant intelligence" and even spawned a new discipline. Electrical signaling in plants was one of the key factors in the birth of "plant neurobiology" (a term used despite the lack of neurons in plants) and today plant researchers are investigating such traditionally non-plant areas as memory, learning, and problem solving.

Despite lacking eyes, plants such as *Arabidopsis* (the model plant) possess at least eleven types of photoreceptors, compared to humans' measly four. This way of thinking has even led to lawmakers in Switzerland setting guidelines designed to protect "the dignity of plants" – whatever that may mean.

"The Venus flytrap, the famous greedy carnivorous plant, [can] still be found in a scattering of swamps in the Southeast….The trap — a highly modified leaf — relies on an action potential, or electrical pulse, to snap shut, a rare power in the floral community….Should an insect land and jostle a hair…'that triggers the first action potential.'" And if, in the next 30 seconds, the luckless visitor touches another hair, wham, the trap snaps shut in a 10th of a second — three times faster than the blink of an eye (*New York Times,* September 15, 2015).

Here are some informative links on this subject, per kind courtesy of Dr. Daniel Chamovitz, former Chair of Plant Sciences at Tel Aviv University:

https://www.youtube.com/watch?v=Qv-iluydZOo&t=2s
https://www.youtube.com/watch?v=ufSRWfrFA-8
https://www.youtube.com/watch?v=36hewUn3KIA&t=3s
https://www.youtube.com/watch?v=DQ39Z7fbO14
https://storypreservation.wordpress.com/2015/09/10/what-a-plant-knows/

Many consider terms like "plant intelligence" and "plant neurobiology" to be metaphorical; they have still been met with a lot of criticism, not the least from Dr. Chamovitz, the renowned research biologist and author of the intriguing book *What A Plant Knows: A Field Guide to the Senses*.

"Do I think plants are smart? I think plants are complex," Chamovitz replied during my interview in his research laboratory in Israel. "Complexity should not be confused with intelligence," he added.

So, while it is useful to describe plants in anthropomorphic terms to communicate ideas, there are limits. The danger is that we end up viewing plants as inferior versions of animals, which completely misses the point.

"Plant scientists are happy to talk about similarities and differences between plant and animal lifestyles when presenting results of plant research to the general public," says Fatima Cvrckova, a plant scientist at Charles University in Prague. "Reliance on animal-based metaphors to describe plants comes with issues. You want to avoid such metaphors, unless you are interested in a usually futile debate about a carrot's ability to feel pain when you bite into it."

Plants are supremely adapted for doing exactly what they need to do. They may lack a nervous system, a brain, and other features we associate with complexity, but they excel in other areas. Chamovitz points out in his book, "light for a plant is much more than a signal; light is food." While plants face many of the same challenges as animals, their sensory requirements are equally shaped by the things that distinguish them: "The rootedness of plants – the fact that they are unmoving – means they actually have to be much more aware of their environment than you or I do."

A Few Basic Benefits to Start With

Aloe: skin bruises and burns heal best with sap
Elderberry: will prevent influenza
Capsicum Peppers: present in pain relief creams, Dr. Pepper, Tabasco sauce
Cranberries: prevent bacteria from planting on the bladder lining (UTI), prevent dental plaque and may have anticancer properties
Chase Tree: prevents premenstrual syndrome; monks used to dampen sexual desires
Garlic: lowers cholesterol but should be avoided before complicated surgery since it may promote bleeding
Ginger: prevents sea sickness and nausea of pregnancy and benefits arthritic conditions
Ginkgo: enhances cerebral and pelvic blood flow
Ginseng: used for centuries to relieve stress, also an aphrodisiac
Milk Thistle: overcomes liver toxins (mushroom poisoning) and hepatitis

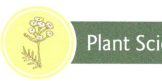

Plant Science Origins...

> "Let food be thy medicine and medicine be thy food."
>
> ~ Hippocrates

Evidence for plants as drugs has been found on a Sumerian clay slab, approximately 5000 years old. It included 12 recipes for drug preparation, referring to over 250 various plants, including poppy, henbane, and mandrake (see https://www.ncbi.nlm.nih.gov/pmc/articles/PMC3358962/#ref2). The Chinese Emperor Shen Ung, circa 2500 BC, used 365 dried plants as medicines. The Indian holy books mention treatment with plants, which are still abundant and used today. Many originated in India, e.g. nutmeg, pepper, clove & curcumin (turmeric), and some are popular as anti-oxidants. The Hebrew Talmud referred to the use of aromatics for important ceremonies and for guarding against the ingestion of toxics while slaughtering potentially dangerous sick animals.

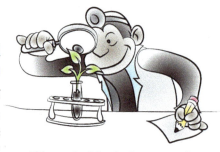

Plant Sciences

[The artist Nicole Cooper and I conceived of these chimp cartoons after it was apparent that chimpanzees would no longer be used in governmental research. We have displayed and acknowledged chimps as a token of their many scientific contributions.]

...Vs Our Modern Diet (how different are we?)

The foods we choose to eat have a direct effect on our health and well-being. Eating whole foods, well-balanced and properly prepared, is vital to maintaining and improving our health. Nutritional science teaches us that choosing the wrong foods, e.g. processed foods, may promote disease. Processed or convenience foods are heavily marketed and are commonly present on most of the shelves in nearly every supermarket today. These high-caloric snacks and manufactured meals are a lucrative business, yet often do little to provide our bodies with the essentials that we need to keep us healthy.

Fresh fruits and vegetables, grains and beans, and grass-fed animal products do provide the more than 1000+ phytonutrients that we regularly need to support our health. Phytonutrients are bioactive compounds (think antioxidants) that supply color and flavor. Antioxidants work to protect our bodies from free radicals, exposure to pollution and the unstable molecules that are produced through metabolism. When it comes to making healthy food choices, consider the many benefits plants offer.

We can now manipulate the DNA of the cacao bean to enhance the taste of chocolate. We can alter the genome of strawberries to make them sweeter and more disease resistant. We can make broccoli resist hot and humid conditions using hybrid methods. These are just a few genetic alterations to improve our food with many more to come.

We hunt for the substances that can boost the human body's ability to stave off disease — mostly from plants. How enzymes convert substances into chemicals the human body needs to function remains a challenge. Some argue that reducing cancer through prevention isn't an option — it's a necessity. (Publication of the molecular structure of the anti-cancer plant-based compound sulforaphane was initially rejected by *Science*, a leading scientific journal; it was eventually published in the *Proceedings of the National Academy of Sciences* in 1992).

The dietary supplements business — comprised of pills and potions made of vitamins, minerals, and herbs that may do little to improve health — has boomed from a $12 billion national industry in 1997 to $22 billion a decade later. Instead we should be consuming plants that have developed thousands of chemicals that act as pesticides or protection against infection. Humans eat as many as 10,000 of these compounds when they chomp on vegetables.

Plant Pigments, pt 1 — what do they tell us?

> "If oranges are called oranges, why aren't lemons called yellows?"
> ~ Unknown

Green color: The spinach family, e.g. asparagus, broccoli, kiwi, green beans, limes, peas, etc., contain the lutein and zeaxanthin carotenoids that help prevent macular degeneration and support healthy tissues, skin and blood.

Orange-ish color: Carrots, pumpkins, and sweet potatoes are an excellent source of Vitamin A. They are also a good source of manganese, copper, Vitamin B5 (pantothenic acid) and Vitamin B6. Additionally, they are a good source for potassium, dietary fiber, Vitamin B1, Vitamin B2, Vitamin C, and phosphorus. Oranges are also an excellent source of Vitamin C. Mashed pumpkin seeds are useful in the treatment and relief of an overactive bladder.

Reddish color: Red apples, pomegranates, raspberries, red cherries, rhubarb, strawberries, and tomatoes all contain the important antioxidants, lycopene and other carotenes. They have been reported to provide anti-inflammatory, anti-cancer and age-related memory benefits and to protect against cancer, especially of the prostate.

Yellowish color: Citrus such as limes, grapefruit and lemons, as well as apricots, peaches, mandarin oranges, mangoes, yellow apples and papayas are a source of Vitamin A, have anti-cancer and heart protective properties, and protect mucous membranes. These inherent colorful plant pigments add much to our well-being.

Mushrooms R Medicine — the good news

> *After years of living in awe of the mysterious fungi, known as Mushrooms — chefs, health enthusiasts, and home cooks alike can't get enough of these rich, delicate morsels*
>
> ~ publisher's description—Paul Stamets, Growing Gourmet and Medicinal Mushrooms

And then there are mushrooms, which in ancient Egypt were reserved for royalty. Romans thought mushrooms conferred strength to warriors.

Today, mushrooms are grown commercially and their benefits are available to all.

The good news is that many mushrooms provide enormous health-promoting benefits, including as a source of iron and Vitamin D. Mushrooms lower cholesterol, help one lose weight, improve cardiovascular health and boost the immune system. There is also evidence that white button mushrooms, such as cremini, remove excess estrogen from circulation, making them helpful for preventing breast cancer. They are also a good source of fiber.

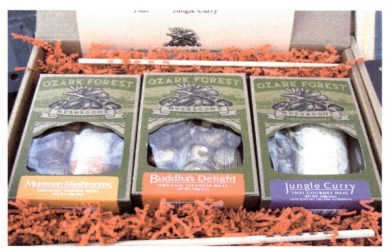

Gourmet mushroom meals (courtesy of author)

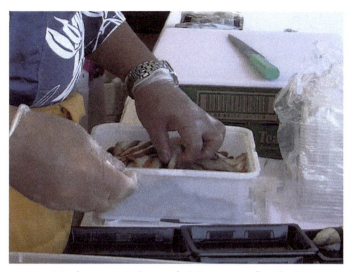

Mushrooms at the market (courtesy of author)

In the foothills of the Himalayas lives a rare Tibetan mushroom. It is more valuable than gold, and more powerful than any drug in western medicine. Ayurvedic, Tibetan and Chinese medical traditions treasured this fungus for centuries. It is considered to be a remarkable cure-all for colds, headaches, infertility and heart problems. It also improves immune system function. Long chain polysaccharides, particularly alpha- and beta-glucan molecules, are primarily responsible for the mushrooms' beneficial effect on the immune system.

The bad news is that there have been recent cases of lethal food poisonings related to eating wild mushrooms. Of the over 10,000 species of mushrooms, only about 50 to 100 are toxic while over 90% of deaths, including the most recent ones, are caused by amatoxins—the collective name of a subgroup of at least eight related toxic compounds found in several genera of poisonous mushrooms and most notably **the death cap.** Unlike many ingested poisons, the toxins are not destroyed by heat, so cooking the poisonous mushrooms does not diminish their danger.

Amandes Phalloides

"When in doubt, throw it out."

An example is the seemingly innocuous "little white mushroom," found in highland tree stumps of Yunnan China, which has suddenly killed many innocent "nibblers" via a silent cardiac toxin which causes abrupt long Q-T intervals. (Excessive barium soil content may be contributory since the deaths often follow monsoons.)

Cordyceps, aka caterpillar fungus

Cordyceps, also called caterpillar fungus or tochukaso, is a favorite of Olympic athletes because it increases strength and endurance and has anti-aging effects. It is a great source for ATP, a high-energy molecule found in every cell. ATP supplies cells with needed energy. The nuclear cell engine is the mitochondria. This important cell organelle has been isolated by George Wu and his team at UConn Health. Wu's research with mitochondria may potentially lead to successful liver transplants. This is a typical example of how different areas of research in plant science are becoming relevant to medical science.

This parasitic mushroom is unique because, in the wild, it grows out of an insect host instead of a plant host. It has long been used in both traditional Chinese and Tibetan medicine. The Cordyceps mushroom has hypoglycemic and possible antidepressant effects, protects the liver and kidneys, increases blood flow, helps normalize cholesterol levels and has been used to treat Hepatitis B. Cordyceps also has antitumor properties. Scientists at the University of Nottingham have been studying this fungus as a potential cancer drug.

More recent studies suggest it also has potent anti-inflammatory characteristics that may be useful for those suffering from resistant asthma, rheumatoid arthritis, renal failure and stroke disorders. New findings indicate that cordycepin acts by a completely different mechanism than currently used anti-inflammatory drugs; thus it is a potential drug for patients for whom the current drugs are ineffective.

The Good & the Bad

Future Potentials

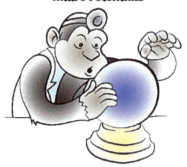

The zeal for food fads and alternative or complementary medicine has spawned increasing use of many exotic health food products. Exposure of travelers to diverse cultural uses of herbal medicines for 'cures' is increasing. However, herbs often contain potential toxins; herbal ingestion always requires microbiologic analysis before it can be recommended for medicinal use.

An example:

This Russian traveler used this one-penny water dispenser to quench her thirst, only to experience marked weight loss. She had ingested the water-borne parasite *Giardia lamblia*. Giardiasis is an infection in the small intestine caused by this microscopic parasite. Giardiasis spreads through contact and is one of the most common causes of waterborne disease in the

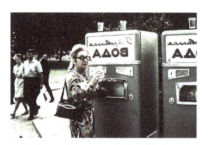

Water dispenser in USSR, late 1960s (courtesy of author)

United States. Symptoms include abdominal cramps, bloating, nausea and watery diarrhea, and the marked weight loss mimics cancer. This condition can be treated by a medical professional. *Giardia lamblia* can be defeated by 9 different plants.

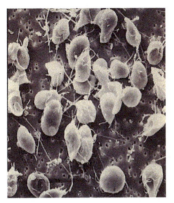 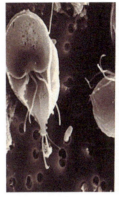 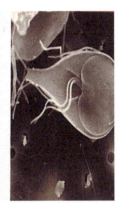

Giardia lamblia *(courtesy of author)*

We are all vulnerable, yet disorders are often overlooked by many. Therefore, we continually strive to expand our clinical judgment. Some parasites are tolerated by humans, but many are not. For instance, most people are not aware that uncooked meat may alter one's immune system, especially if the animal product was derived from an animal that had ingested or had been injected with steroids.

A gourmet steak tartare meal of uncooked beef mixed with raw egg may potentially contain *Taenia saginata*, a beef tapeworm, which can be detected by the colonic passage of the proglottid segments.

A restaurant's four-star rating may be changed by the ingestion of steak tartare and converted into the four oral suckers of this cestode. Rare pork meat exposures may produce delayed bizarre calcified implants in the brain, ribs and bone, long after the menu's content can be recalled.

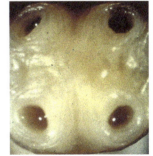

Tapeworm head *(courtesy of author)*

On the contrary, pomegranate seeds, quinacrine, and oleum resin from bark are plant-derived medications that may destroy parasites. Cestode therapy acts by weakening the worm's muscular holdings to the host.

Still another example of plant-derived medicine is the powdered wormwood, *Artemisia absinthium*, combined with the green hulls of black walnuts (http://www.kitchendoctor.com/herbs/black_walnut.php), as a traditional treatment for parasites. A recent study at the University of Washington suggests that a different species of wormwood, *Artemisia annua*, (http://www.cancersalves.com/botanical_approaches/individual_

herbs/wormwood.html) the famed anti-malarial herb that is also effective in many parasitic formulas, has significant anti-cancer properties as well (http://www.cancerplants.com/herb_news/herbal_news.html).

Many helminthic infections are worldwide burdens. A sample is illustrated here:

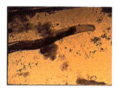

Strongyloides worm (courtesy of author)

Some humans stock their medicine cabinets with futuristic nourishments. Touting the use of insects as alternative wholesome "food" reminds me of my friend Dr. Benjamin Milder's delightful poem:

> Still, diets made of locusts and wild honey must be viable cause they were John's sustenance—it says so in the Bible
>
> ~ Benjamin Milder, MD

The mulberry tree caterpillar (the silkworm) provides us with ultra-strong spider fibers after voraciously eating the leaves to sustain its remarkable metabolism, as illustrated here:

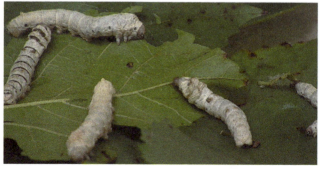

Silk-producing caterpillars (courtesy of author)

Some years ago, it was falsely reported that a medication derived from apricot seeds (Laetrile) could cure cancer. This resulted in a mad dash of patients and/or their families to Mexico where the drug was available. A few years later, Laetrile was shown by scientists to be ineffective. Many other obtuse but lucrative ventures continue to mislead desperate families. The ongoing search for phytochemicals, such as the highly successful Madagascar chemotherapeutic agents from Rose Periwinkle—the source of vinblastine and vincristine—has proven to be highly effective for the treatment of childhood leukemia and non-Hodgkin's lymphoma. This discovery of effective plant-derived cancer drugs has motivated the National Institutes of Health (NIH) to expand their focus on phytogeographic agents.

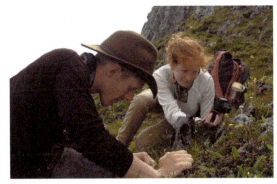
Researchers in Tibet (courtesy of author)

Some green teas are said to prevent cancers, yet very few people ever consider the potential adverse reactions to tea.

Popular teas such as kitchen-made "Kombucha mushroom" have been associated with acute metabolic acidosis and aspergillus contamination; and veno-occlusive liver disease and death have followed the ingestion of germander *(Teucrium chamaedrys),* gordolobo and *symphytum* (comfrey) teas due to intrinsic pyrrolizidine alkaloids. Chaparral, derived from the desert shrub creosote, has caused fulminant hepatic failure.

Drinking or smoking the resin of boiled Jimson Weed seeds results in severe anticholinergic toxicity associated with brain dysfunction. Herbal Paraguay tea causes bizarre behavioral abnormalities.

Medical Students– *"Would you have questioned your patient about consumption of unusual teas?"*

Patients – *"Would you have shared this information with your doctor?"*

With the explosion of Internet-based ads, many herbs are promoted as "digestive aids, stress relievers, weight loss agents and aphrodisiacs." These are largely unregulated, which is a concern. Drinking herbal infusions containing benzaldehyde and cinnamoyl has produced hepato-renal failure, bleeding, and intravascular coagulopathy (D.I.C.). Chinese herbal use, resulting in a kidney disorder, may be a clue to Fanconi Syndrome or the recent Balkan interstitial nephropathy epidemic, induced by toxic aristolochic acid, contained in that magic bottle sold door-to-door.

Analgesic and cardiotonic preparations containing highly toxic aconite alkaloids have produced tetraplegia, ventricular irregularity and death. Other root concoctions such as Konzo contain cyanogens present in **unboiled** cassava roots. Bonesetter's herbs, for example 'Zheng Gu Shui' and 'Tieh Ta Yao Gin,' are commonly prescribed to reduce post-traumatic pain and swelling: each contains a putative dermatitis allergen, *Myrrh*. The 'medicinal' use of glycyrrhetinic acid **(licorice)** may lead to 'essential' hypertension. The recent popularity of 'squalene' has produced shark oil pneumonitis.

Suspecting only occupational sources for heavy metal poisoning may overlook the contamination of many health food products as well as NSAID products, steroids and microorganisms. These associations become subtle diagnostic crystal-ball challenges for clinicians who properly assess modern travelers, expatriates and herbal enthusiasts for latent exposures.

What Your Ancestors Knew

While no single food, food group, or supplement available today can guarantee perfect health, our ancestors do offer some guidance. The historic and wildly popular 1800s cookbook *The Prudent Housewife, or Compleat English Cook* contained directions for "Marketing, Roasting, Boiling, Stewing, Baking, Rules to Be Observed for Pickling, Preserving, and A Treasury of Valuable Medicine, For The Cure of Every Disorder," with instructions not only for preparing daily meals but also identifying and curing illnesses. With a very long title, this book guided the middle-class family as they relied on the prescribed ingredients to treat measles, deafness and coughs, etc. Most people didn't go to the doctor; instead, they relied on self-diagnosis, self-treatment and traditional wisdom to take care of common ailments.

While we're less likely to treat a sprain with a warm vinegar soak, followed with a paste of stale beer grounds, oatmeal and hog's lard, the treatment for an earache with "the smoke of tobacco blown into the ear" was indeed fashionable and formidable. Today, there are suggestions everywhere to maintain good health. When we get a cold or an aching shoulder, we rely on our doctors to cure us. What we seem to overlook is that many maladies can be prevented by making different life choices, including diet or treatment with more natural remedies. Taking an active role in the maintenance of our health and the best treatment for any disorders should be the goal of every individual and health care professional.

This eBook is intended to provide a supportive and more natural, yet limited, approach to healing and to provide guidance for the curious and the concerned.

The Lessons of Patient Histories (be patient)

Taking a history from a patient is a skill necessary for all doctors before and after examinations, provides a valuable record of the patient/doctor interaction, and provides the best and most rapid pathway to diagnosis and treatment.

The doctor might ask a series of questions of the patient, such as the nature of the complaint, details of onset, pain level (if any), contributing factors such as the evolution of the symptoms; history of treatment(s) and responses; and other health history, including past diseases, drug allergies, sexual preferences, surgical complications, drug and alcohol use, herbal or supplement use, over-the-counter drug use and family history.

> "Sadly, today physicians rarely focus on the patient's story, usurped by a need for reports, time compressions, and technological foci. I believe a physician's focus on a patient may best computers every time."
>
> ~ author's interview of *American Journal of Gastroenterology* editor

Physicians should also inquire about exposures, occupation, pets, and hobbies or ongoing interests. It is understood that a diagnosis as revealed in the patient's history needs to be identified. Often the history alone does reveal a diagnosis, and it begins with establishing rapport with patients who invariably need reassurance.

Our theme of "a diagnosis is easy, as long as you think of it" (Soma Weiss) must be always kept in mind! Recall that it takes probing, practice, patience, understanding and listening with a third ear to make a useful diagnosis. A typical example is the following case.

The Yale Swim Team worked out in Florida during their spring break. After eating a luncheon that included a well-cooked fish sandwich, the team captain became violently ill with mouth paresthesia, "an abnormal sensation, typically tingling or prickling (think pins and needles) where hot tasted cold and cold tasted hot."

Some weakness in his swallowing, a perplexing symptom, caused his prompt return to New Haven and my immediate care. I began taking his history while probing for clues. Was it early polio or perhaps multiple sclerosis (MS), a disease in which the immune system eats away at the protective covering of nerves? My assessment, however, convinced me that the totality of symptoms did not indicate MS.

The patient's family was understandably worried. Was it possible that the young swim captain was suffering from event histrionics? Were his pronounced physical symptoms the result of dramatic inadequate feelings and hyperventilation? Was the pressure of the swim team's success causing an emotional overreaction? While symptoms can include near paralysis and difficulty swallowing, nothing in his history suggested an emotionally dramatic event.

The diagnostic reasoning process continued as I inquired about his activities prior to the onset of symptoms. He was able to describe his lunch, and I was then able to make the diagnosis readily upon probing the crucial question: "does hot taste cold and does cold taste hot?"

The culprit, the fish, had produced…Ciguatera Poisoning, of course! The problem

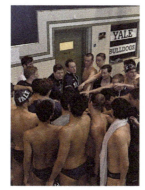

Yalies at spring training in Florida (courtesy of author)

had begun at the luncheon table; the otherwise healthy young man had enjoyed a barracuda sandwich. Ciguatera poisoning was caused by eating the toxic-laden fish.

Amberjack, sea bass, red snapper and Spanish mackerel live in coral reefs. Ciguatera toxins tend to accumulate in predator fish, such as the barracuda and other carnivorous reef fish, because they eat other fish that consume toxin-producing algae (dinoflagellates) that live in these coral reef waters.

Ciguatera toxins are harmless to fish but poisonous to humans. The toxin is odorless and tasteless. It is heat-resistant, so cooking does not destroy the toxin. Eating a ciguatera-contaminated tropical or subtropical predatory fish will poison the person who eats it. An immediate and robust response was forthcoming. Reassurance followed for the family that recovery was imminent and that he would again swim free-style during the next collegiate meet. Mystery solved. Yale swimmers won the subsequent New England Conference!

Many "food-hardy" people are tempted to indulge in robust "treats." Here are a few for the adventurous traveler as samplers.

Should one dare consume the prized meat of a bear during a Canadian summer canoeing trip? A graduate student who developed high fever, muscular pains and near coma required air evacuation transfer by the Royal Canadian Police. The extracted history pointed to our diagnosis of trichinosis, despite the diverting symptoms of cardiac irregularity and thrombophlebitis being prominent in this student's physical signs. The medical history, which included that he had eaten slaughtered bear meat, merited his physician's pride in the resulting recovery.

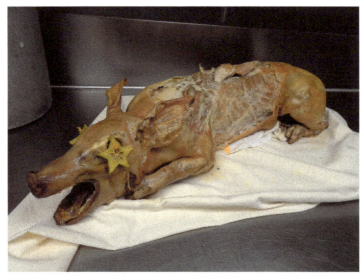

After a pig roast (courtesy of author)

One must be alert to "special" food gatherings. Try to diagnose this celebratory pig roast event, interrupted by several sick children who experienced the sudden onset of weakness, nausea, vomiting, severe abdominal pain and near collapse. The prompt recognition of this syndrome by an emergency room resident, who asked the proper roasting temperature of the pig, averted a near tragedy.

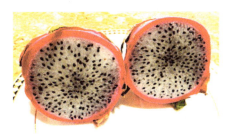

Dragon fruit (courtesy of author)

The dragon fruit (used to decorate the pig's eyes) did not cause this episode. Instead, the treacherous "Pig Bel," a syndrome of necrotizing enteritis due to *Clostridium perfringens*, was the culprit. Intense roasting for less than four hours often invites this unexpected ingredient as a dangerous bacterial toxin that may be fatal if not recognized and treated promptly. Other ingested food products to be aware of include soft cheeses and some seafood types. The latter may contain methyl mercury, a modern scourge of today's contamination sources.

Today, there are competing drugstores at every corner and crossroad. Yet before pharmaceutical companies and medicine became big business and changed the way we treat illness, there were plants, along with people (mostly women) who knew how to use them.

Illnesses, common ailments and even life-threatening diseases were cured with homegrown remedies. Tonics, teas, tinctures, seeds and poultices were used to cure disease, boost energy, cure a cold, relieve a backache, drain an abscess, and settle an upset stomach. Pregnancies were interrupted by special herbals.

Since biblical times, we humans have used plants to help us heal and improve our quality of life. And the journey, a sort of huge 'clinical trial,' has been an interesting one! This medical journey, however, has been burdened with many theories and more than a few hoaxes. Recognizing individuals who introduce new methods and are true inventive pioneers, yet who have been belittled by their jealous peers, often requires our own objectivity. Such is the case when I became 'hooked on Hooke' while library browsing.

> **The art of healing comes from nature, not from the physician. Therefore, the physician must start from Nature, with an open mind.**
> ~ Paracelsus

Hooked on Hooke — & other pioneers & key inventions

More than 350 years have passed since Robert Hooke, a true Renaissance man, authored the best-seller *Micrographia*.

Micrographia was the first book to illustrate insects, plants, etc., as seen through microscopes. Published in 1665 by the Royal Society, it became the first scientific bestseller. It included astonishing images of leeches in vinegar, a flea in finely drawn detail, the minutia of a mosquito, a spider with six eyes, gnats, pores in petrified wood, and diamonds in flint, as well as the early-recognized cork cell. This masterpiece of scientific observation became the forerunner of crystallography (see the Titan Krios Microscope), planetary exploration, fossil archeology, the anatomy of insects, and even a method for the production of artificial silk. Published in 1665 and weighing nearly three pounds, this historically significant book introduced the world to the new science of microscopy. Adding light and focus, Hooke improved the microscope and immediately observed the smallest and previously hidden details of the natural world.

> " By the help of Microscopes, there is nothing so small, as to escape our enquiry; hence there is a new visible World discovered to the understanding. "
>
> ~ Robert Hooke

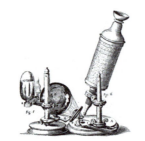

Compound microscope (from Robert Hooke, Micrographia, 1665)

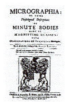

Micrographia by Robert Hooke (1665)

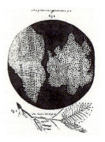

Cork cell (from Robert Hooke, Micrographia, 1665)

Reportedly, Hooke made a startling discovery while studying the bark of a cork tree: it was comprised of tiny structures or building blocks. These microscopic "building blocks" reminded him of the small individual rooms in a Christian monastery, a.k.a. "cells." That afternoon, Robert Hooke coined the phrase "plant cells" and introduced the world to the basic building blocks of all living things. Robert Hooke had one of the most creative minds in the history of science; he regularly provoked and amazed skeptics.

Hooke's seminal discovery of the feasibility of microscopy, soon to become a great engine of research, is matched by his intuitive correlations with other phenomena. The laws of optics, combustion, and the behavior of liquids in capillary tubes, all of which he formulated and outlined in his book, were seldom subsequently challenged.

The meticulous drawings and accurate observations of this energetic 28-year-old fledgling scientist were recognized by many of the original purchasers of the book, who proudly joined Samuel Pepys (an English naval administrator and Member of Parliament best known for his "Diary" accounts of great events, such as the Great Plague of London, the Second Dutch War, and the Great Fire of London) in sensing its unique qualities.

Despite his incredible achievements, not everyone was a fan. Henry Oldenburg, Secretary of the Royal Society, often omitted Hooke's name from recorded comments and rightful priority credits. Their intensifying disputes caused Hooke to call Oldenburg a "trafficker in intelligence." Even the Royal Society caused Hooke dismay when his honorarium was never paid (despite polite reminders), and eventually the Council demanded he deduct a grant pledge from his meager salary.

Is it any wonder that Hooke's digestive tract required this "tailoring" of his "stomach?": he would partake of one meal and one dish, which he would supplement with powdered silver, syrup of poppy seed, and liberal use of bleeding with cuppings, which was the famous ancillary treatment of clysters.

Despite these problems, Hooke was able to perceive and predict the future application of his nearly one thousand inventions. While always dressed in his personally chosen long fashions, sewn by himself, Hooke gregariously interacted in coffee shops with many notables, but was never able to sustain wide recognition of his work. Hooke died a feeble, depressed, reclusive man, despite his legacies to science and also his personal wealth, found dormant in an iron chest, of several thousand pounds of earned silver and gold coins (apparently for late payments as a surveyor and architect after the London Fire in 1666).

And then there was Sir Isaac……

Isaac Newton

While the apple falling onto his head is surely a myth, Newton came to understand that the force that caused the apple to come crashing to the ground also related to the moon falling toward the earth: i.e. gravity.

> "If I have seen further it is by standing on the shoulders of giants."
> ~ Isaac Newton, in a letter to Robert Hooke, 1676

Despite having much to be proud of in his own life, Newton wasn't necessarily a happy nor a self-confident man. Shortly after being elected to the Royal Society, Newton developed a rivalry with the more famous member, Robert Hooke, whom he referred to as "this miserable philosopher." Newton's remarks about standing on the shoulders of giants was actually very unpleasant in regard to Robert Hooke, a bent, shriveled and crooked man. The jealousy ran deep: Newton may have waited for Hooke's death before publishing his dormant *Opticks* and then failed to acknowledge Hooke's prior work. Some hinted that Newton had a nervous breakdown.

Similarly, Newton disagreed with William Briggs, ophthalmologist and physician to King William III. The mathematician waited 21 years before publishing his *Nova visionis theoria*, then free of a co-contributor.

Nicholas Culpeper influenced many during his four decades of life, popularizing astrological herbalism: "he that would know the reason of the operation of the Herbs, must look up as high as the stars." His famous book *The English Physician* warranted 40 editions.

Franz Mesmer

For years, the German physician Franz Mesmer had been making headlines with his controversial theory of animal and plant magnetism. He touted the idea that everything in the universe, including the human body, was governed by a "majestic fluid" that could become imbalanced, causing illness. Hypnotizing members of the French Society, Dr. Mesmer claimed to have magnetized certain trees that could then "cure" those imbalanced patients. Introspective and wealthy societies flocked to Mesmer's salon. Frances, King of France, appointed Benjamin Franklin, Chairman of the French Royal Commission on Mesmerism, to investigate these claims.

Franklin's final analysis: "imagination and false suggestion" was key to the popularity of mesmerism in France. Franklin further indicated that his own gout was uncured and that other Commission members' complaints also were unrelieved by Mesmer. Franklin stated: "He's the best physician that knows the worthlessness of most medicines."

> "This young woman is in urgent need of assistance of Franz Anton Mesmer! Mesmer!"
> ~ from the movie *Doctor Strange* (2016)

Mozart, a close friend of Mesmer's, used magnets to cure one of his characters in *Cosi Fan Tutte*. The magnet theory attracted an enthusiastic following (the rich and then famous) between 1780 and 1850 and continued to have some influence until the end of the century. One of those entranced by the theory was Dr. Joseph-Ignace Guillotin who espoused the theory that "the instant beheading" of his machine, the guillotine, "saved the onset of the victim's torture."

How ironic that current scientists now rely on powerful magnets within CT and PET scanners, radiating laser beams, ultrasonic probes, current levitation physics and the like for breakthroughs in their newest discoveries. Today, mesmerism, as it came to be known, is almost entirely forgotten. Although it is still practiced as a form of alternative medicine in some countries, magnetic practices are not fully recognized as part of medical science. Dr. Mesmer, however, is well remembered as the forerunner of the practice of hypnotism and was the first to urge vaccination.

Leeches, past & present—and other treatments

Leeches have been used for centuries to treat a wide range of diseases. In 1837, St. Bartholomew's Hospital is credited with using no less than 96,300 leeches to treat patients. The prominent influential French physician François Joseph Victor Broussais supported the "hirudinea-mania" (leech-excitement) that necessitated the importation of 42 million leeches in France and in the U.S. A land leech can be removed by hand, since they do not burrow into the skin or leave the head in the wound. A sore develops and lasts for about a week.

> "The government has lent its seal of approval to marketing an age-old medical device — leeches."
> ~ Associated Press, June 28th 2004

While often viewed as a creepy and gruesome sight, "There was hardly a French belly which had not given nourishment to these blood suckers." Subsequently, the leeches' local salivary anticoagulant, hirudin, was made into its recombinant form, r-hirudin, in 1991, and is now widely used to inhibit blood clotting (intravascular coagulopathy).

Surprisingly, the application of these living, segmented worms to the skin has made a comeback in the treatment of hemochromatosis (a rare iron disorder in which the body simply loads too much iron), polycythemia (an abnormally increased concentration of hemoglobin in the blood), pulmonary edema, various autoimmune disorders and toxic poisoning. Blood-letting seems to have been validated by modern studies. Unfortunately, not all discoveries have been as beneficial to the promotion of health.

The Clyster (enema) was particularly fashionable from the 17th through the 19th centuries. In high society, enemas became enormously popular, with some aristocratic hypochondriacs taking several scented enemas a day.

Included in the diverse treatments of near drowning was insufflating tobacco smoke into clysters as a foundation or "fundiments."

Soon thereafter, Sir John Harrington's invention of the water closet undoubtedly endeared him to Queen Elizabeth and further contributed to the discontinuance of clysters by her subjects.

Still more magical concoctions were touted by a few industrious druggists. *A Pharmacopoeia Londinensis of 1618* listed use of mummy dust, human and pigeon excrement, stag penis and a unicorn's horn. At a later date, *Beehive's Materia Medica* recommended other concoctions with oil of scorpions, troches of vipers, crabs' eyes and dragon blood.

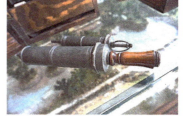
Lewis and Clark's original clyster (courtesy of author)

The nostrums of old consistently attracted many medical messiahs, exemplified by the quackery of A.J. White, residing in New York in 1883. The Shaker-Village-Made remedy of "Pain Kill," consisting of 10-30 drops of sugar water, was given every half hour until the "digestive morbus" was relieved. Analysis would have disclosed its base of opium, camphor, witch hazel and alcohol.

Another New York State basement-derived inventive treatment for an epidemic of cholera became "Pepto-Bismol." Its inventor could hardly envision its later successful use in treatment of other digestive illnesses such as travelers' diarrhea and helicobacter pylori infection or common indigestion.

William Osler & Harvey Cushing

The painting *The Four Doctors* (1906) by John Singer Sargent depicts Dr. William H. Welch (the first Dean of Johns Hopkins Medical School), Dr. William Osler (extraordinary Clinician of Medicine—responsible for training by clinical observations), Dr. William S. Halsted (pathologist who set up the intern/resident postgraduate training program) and Dr. Howard A. Kelly (obstetrician). These were named the Founding Fathers of Johns Hopkins School of Medicine. Dr. Osler created the first residency program for specialty training of physicians, and he was the first to bring medical students out of the lecture hall and to the bedside for clinical training.

> "Listen to your patient, he is telling you the diagnosis"
> ~ Sir William Osler

Dr. Osler has been labelled the "Father of Modern Medicine." His greatest influence on medicine, however, was to insist that students learn from seeing and talking to patients, as well as by taking good notes; he also established the higher medical residency. This idea spread across the English-speaking world and remains in place today in most teaching hospitals.

His best-known saying presages the later quotation by Soma Weiss which emphasizes the importance of listening to the patient and taking a good history: "A diagnosis is easy, as long as you think of it." Sir William Osler died at the age of 70 in 1919, yet his renowned demeanor lives on, beyond his first edition of the *Practice of Medicine* in 1897.

Dr. Harvey Cushing (1869-1939) was a close friend and colleague of Dr. Osler. In 1929 Dr. Harvey Cushing won the Pulitzer Prize for his biography of Sir William Osler.

By all accounts, Dr. Harvey Cushing was a brilliant brain surgeon. Through his research on the pituitary gland, he became one of the founders of endocrinology, and probably thereafter best known for describing Cushing's Disease. Cushing attracted Ivan Pavlov and many other notables. The Medical Historical Library at Yale includes a famous Mason Jar containing a steak with Pavlov's signature, which he inscribed with Cushing's early Bove electrosurgical knife after watching Cushing perform a procedure. Many other memorabilia in the room reflect the serious scientific approach to the many vagaries of Cushing's pioneering neurosurgery.

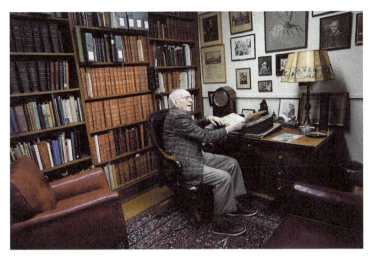
Author at his desk in Harvey Cushing's former office (courtesy of author)

This author was privileged to reside in Cushing's office for 10 years as Board Chairman of the Cushing/Whitney Medical Library Associates.

Olaus Rudbeck, Joseph Lister, & a Few More

Reflect now on still other pioneers, beginning with Olaus Rudbeck, who impacted our subsequent welfare. Forgotten and often misunderstood and unheeded, these early leaders groped for the pre-science of digestion and patient care.

While still a 20-year-old student, Rudbeck (1630-1702) made keen observations of women dressing a calf. This led him to tracing chyle from the mesentery to the thoracic duct. Olaus Rudbeck the Elder, as he was known, was a Swedish scientist and writer, Professor of Medicine at Uppsala University, Rector administrator at the same university, producer of over 7,000 herbarium plates, bridge engineer and craftsman.

He recognized the hazard of tobacco smoking and remains a pioneer in understanding the lymphatic system. His findings and research in the area of human anatomy were supported by Queen Christina of Sweden. While Professor of Medicine, he built an arena-like *Theatrum* in order to carry out dissections of human cadavers for the benefit of students.

During and before the early 18th century, appalling numbers of deaths were occurring following surgeries. While working in Pasteur's Laboratory, Joseph Lister recognized the suppuration of microorganisms. His preventive application of carbolic acid was not acceptable to most physicians. Even his students, in disbelief, failed to attend his classes. Sir Joseph Lister, Bt. (1827-1912) became a British surgeon and pioneer of antiseptic surgery. In Wikipedia, he is shown "spraying phenol over a patient." Only near his death was he honored for his germ theory, and for his achievements in sterilizing operative instruments, and thus preventing infections, while advancing abdominal surgery.

Illuminating innovative inventions have occurred through the centuries. The "pinna," a vomiting feather, was said to relieve the Roman banqueter replete with gluttony. When necessary, the hapless patient was suspended in a swinging bed to induce vomiting. Lead and coin-silver tubes were occasionally used. Monks secretly passed flexible whale bones, tufted with horsehair or linen, called "The Magenkratzers." These instruments presumably gave relief for toothaches, apoplexy, drunkenness and other ills afflicting the distinguished men of Royalty. Appreciative fees and gratuitous grants were difficult to obtain, which sounds similar to today's funding difficulties.

This 18th-century booklet below chronicles a progressive invention, although initially crude and rigid. It was written by <u>Edward Jukes</u>, Esquire, who vehemently declared and defended his invention of a flexible stomach tube, and illustrates the invariable battles for recognition while many inventors were scorned or totally ignored.

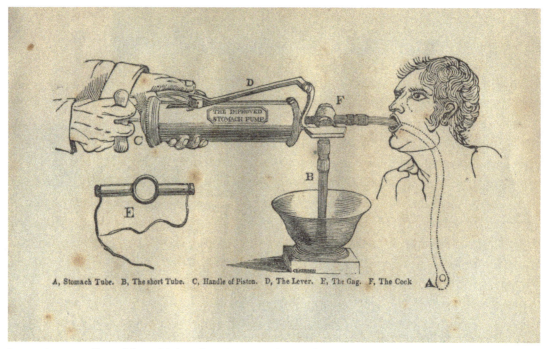

Stomach pump (from Edward Jukes, Esquire, Remarks on the Invention of the Stomach-pump, *1832)*

Among the instruments Sanctorius (1561-1636), the Italian physician and physiologist, invented was the trocar—for removing excess water from the abdomen and chest—and catheter for removing kidney stones.

Abdominal paracentesis also has a long and competitive history, exemplified by Santorio Santorio (called Santorius), an inventive professor of Padua who kept his metal trocar invention for treatment of dropsy a very guarded secret. His students were only permitted to view the ascitic fluid after extraction from the hidden draped abdomen.

Scultetus advocated an abdominal binder to maintain the intraabdominal status, while others inserted wicks for continuous abdominal drainage. An abrupt rapid fluid withdrawal initiated occasional adverse physiologic changes affecting the reno-vascular system. A devised abdominal pressurized-corset device allayed these adverse reactions.

Some confirmed their creativity and ingenuity by fashioning challenges for the US Patent Office.

Others warranted a tribute for ingenuity when this "Tapeworm Trap" patent was granted & authorized when seemingly indicated. These early instruments were later succeeded by more flexible fiber optic instruments, relaying computerized digital images to better survey occult mucosal lesions. Recent robotic laparoscopic surgery now treats the entire hepatobiliary and genitourinary systems using microscopic dissections, thus often relieving patients of prolonged postoperative discomfort.

A Dutch inventor attempted earlier to traverse the gut by a motorized intestinal capsule, conveyed along on its track-like string.

Thereafter, small wireless capsules were developed that capture nearly 1,000 images per minute, detecting small and often obscure vascular bleeding sites and hidden tumors in the digestive tract. Wireless commands now guide the capsule's rotations and directions. A new mucosal and surface optical system uses laser/fluorescence and defines neoplastic abnormalities without a biopsy.

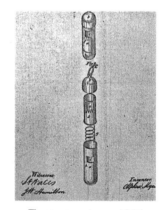

Tapeworm trap, 1854 picture at US Patent Office (courtesy of author)

The ongoing panoramic reviews of discoveries leading to medical applications often omit many worthy persons' laudable achievements. A scrolling list of prominent innovations:

    Babbage's first analytical computing machine, 1833
    Helmholtz's Ophthalmoscope, 1851
    Mendel describes importance of heredity, 1865
    Lister's anti-sepsis solution, 1857
    Tesla makes first AC motor, 1887
    Roentgen discovers X Rays, 1895

Curie discovers radium activity, 1898
Einthoven describes use of EKG, 1903
Metchnikoff's Nobel Prize for immunology and phagocytosis, 1905
Ehrlich uses aniline dyes and discovers salvarsan, 1905
Braggs develops x-ray diffraction to determine crystal structure, 1912
Banting and Best discover the value of insulin; only one received the Nobel prize, 1922
Fleming discovers penicillin, 1928
Bloch and Purcell independently develop MRI, 1946
Lederberg at Yale discovers with Tatum the sexuality of bacteria, 1946
Shockley develops the junction transistor, 1948
Gabor invents holography, 1950
Watson and Crick deduce the structure of DNA, 1953
Townes designs Maser, 1953
Cesium Laser Clock, accuracy one second in 50 million years, 1955
Yale's Palades discovers ribosomes, 1956
Maiman discovers Laser, 1960
Cormack and Hounsfield independently develops CAT scan, 1963
First heart transplant, 1967
Rohrer develops scanning tunneling microscope, showing atoms, 1981
Buck detects Fullerene-60, 1990
Gene defects defined, 1993
Nematode C. Elegans sequenced, 1998
Global explosion of molecular biology, gene expressions and stem cell research, 1990s

Other inventions with unique and innovative applications continue to advance medical therapy. They include the hyperbaric pressure chamber, cardioverters, implantable defibrillators, angioplasty catheters (replacing aortic valves without thoracotomy), Greenfield blood clot stoppers (now being abandoned), laparoscopic "band-aid" instruments, and advancing wireless gastrointestinal viewing capsules.

> He that invents a machine augments the power of man and the well-being of mankind.
> ~ Henry Ward Beecher

Thus, we witness a few vignettes of the incredible inventiveness of many with plant scientists liberally borrowing unique applications. Visionaries such as Robert Hooke and others were rarely acknowledged. Their lives were often replete with frustrations and surrounded by jealous colleagues, yet many remained committed insatiably to their noble tasks.

Peter Raven — a note of wisdom

Peter H. Raven, Ph.D., is a world-renowned botanist and avid conservationist who served for 46 years as President of the Missouri Botanical Garden. In 2000, the American Society of Plant Taxonomists established the Peter Raven Award in his honor to be conferred to authors with outstanding contributions in plant taxonomy.

His wisdom here: "Plants, we've grown up with them. We've been around for about two million years, depending on when you start the clock ticking, and we've lived in a world of plants. They support us in every way, from food to medicine to clothing, and their beauty refreshes our souls, and orients us in a world which, without them, would be dull and humdrum and uninteresting, and not worth living in. Small wonder that they formed such a large part of our inspiration for art. That they fill such a necessary place in our lives. We're part of the living world and plants are one very important way of reminding us of our connection."

Plant Pigments, pt 2

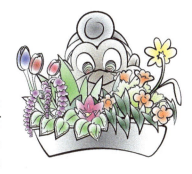

Pigments are responsible for many of the beautiful colors we see in the plant world. From the lush green of photosynthesizing plants to the deep purple of Concord grapes, Nature entices us to notice her bounty. Color plays a multitude of roles in the natural world, used to entice, to camouflage, and to signal harvest time and the change of seasons, from the first green of spring to the brilliant reds and golds of the fall leaves.

Biological pigments are produced by living organisms. They can be found in many plants, including fruits, vegetables, and flowers. Bacteria are colored by pigments. All biological pigments selectively absorb certain wavelengths of light while reflecting others.

Green plants contain the pigment, chlorophyll, that absorbs certain light wavelengths within the visible light spectrum and then decomposes in bright sunlight. Plants constantly synthesize chlorophyll and replenish it. During the fall, as part of their preparation for winter, deciduous plants stop producing chlorophyll, which allows the vivid colors of fall leaves to emerge as yellow and red pigments because of its absence.

Chlorophyll is used as a green dye in commercially processed food, toothpaste, soaps, and cosmetics. A study released in September 2013 determined that compounds containing chlorophyll might help suppress hunger.

Plant pigments exist in a wide variety of forms, some with highly complex and large structures. Over 600 naturally occurring carotenoid structures have been identified, as well as over 7000 biological pigments such as chlorophyll T. These are colored organic molecules which owe their color to the presence of unsaturated bonds.

Photosynthesis — plant energy

The emerging knowledge of photosynthesis is now disclosing electron movements of attosecond range. Shortly after the Nobelist Ahmed Zewail used laser spectrometry, the chemical energy to provide organic matter was revealed. A network of proteins apparently controlled photosynthesis via chlorophyll. That guided the channeled energy towards the reactive center, absorbing and emitting light in a few femtoseconds. The resulting surplus energy within the chlorophyll is then dissipated, emitting light with its heat.

Photosynthesis occurs when plant leaves convert water and minerals from soil, carbon dioxide from the air (which we deliver), and chemical energy stored in special cell membranes to produce energy. The sun pushes the process along and turns the combination into glucose, which becomes the energy plants need to grow.

> " *A big tree seemed even more beautiful to me when I imagined thousands of tiny photosynthesis machines inside every leaf.* "
>
> ~ Cynthia Kenyon, Biologist

Plant leaves contain chlorophyll which makes the leaves green and traps the energy from the sun so the plants can use it as needed. When plants take carbon dioxide from the air, they release oxygen, which humans and all animals require. We actively release carbon dioxide, which the plants need—which further displays Nature's speed, ingenuity and efficiency. Plant scientists are further defining the many silent plant controls through microscopic examinations, just as Robert Hooke caused wonderment as he carefully examined various objects.

Every leaf has multiple macroscopic openings called stomata. These closable air pores on the leaf undersurface are on double duty: they monitor moisture evaporation that brings more moisture and nutrients from the roots; and they bring in carbon dioxide to the leaf lamina for the photosynthesis process. They also govern control of the plant's water needs by alternately opening or closing. Guard Cells govern this process. It is now known that sodium fluxes with osmotic alteration occur silently through this barometric-like control. Grasses have stomata that are less kidney shaped, are linear in distribution, and are very efficient in dealing with our global climate changes.

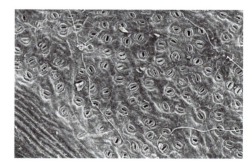

Leaf stomata (courtesy of author)

Plants also need nitrogen to help them grow, phosphorus for strong roots, and potassium to make fruit or vegetables. Even if the use of "night soil" (human excreta) as fertilizer has contributed to the widespread incidence of global parasitism, these soil elements are the pure gifts of Nature's recycling.

These complexities of plant growth are the foundation of a long-favorite human creation…

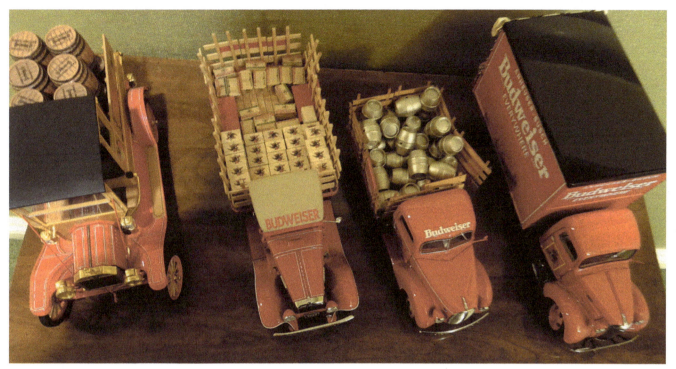

Beer distribution (courtesy of author)

Beer — as old as civilization

After water and tea, beer is the third most widely consumed beverage in the world. It is also our oldest alcoholic beverage. Archaeologists credit beer, both the production and consumption, as a significant factor in the creation of civilization. Early writings have much to say about the laws concerning the production and distribution of beer.

> *He was a wise man who invented beer.*
> ~ Plato

The "Hymn to Ninkasi," the ancient Mesopotamian goddess of beer, served as both a prayer and as a method of remembering the recipe for brewing beer in a culture with few literate people. Written down around 1800 BCE and inscribed on a tablet, it reminded brewers that *"Ninkasi, you are the one who soaks the malt in a jar…"*

Nearly 5000 years ago, workers in the city of Uruk (modern day Iraq) were paid by their employers in beer as well as grains.

During the construction of the Egyptian pyramids, workers were given a large daily ration of beer along with onions, which served as both refreshment and nutrition.

Brewing, which involves the fermentation of starches, mainly began with malted barley and wheat, and was flavored with hops, which acts as a natural preservative.

The fermentation process causes a natural carbonation effect, although this is often removed during processing and replaced with forced carbonation. While all beers vary in their nutritional and alcohol content, all rely on the yeast, *Saccharomyces cerevisiae*, to produce antioxidant substances that prevent oxidation of other molecules.

Brewer's yeast is known to be a rich source of nutrients, and beer can in fact contain significant amounts of necessary nutrients, including magnesium, selenium, potassium, chromium and B vitamins. If consumed in moderation, evidence suggests that beer can increase good cholesterol. One beer a day keeps kidneys healthy and can protect against renal stones. Other benefits include increased levels of Vitamin B while elevated levels of silicon in beer can contribute to higher bone density. Beer may also aid in a restful sleep. However, drinking excessive beer alone may deprive one of Vitamin B1 (thiamine), may also induce cardiac failure, and may result in the massive edema of Beri-Beri deficiency.

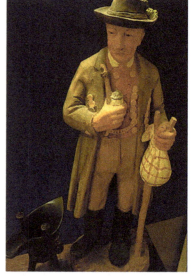
Biermeister (courtesy of author)

So don't plan on getting all your nutrients from beer…unless you're a monk.

In Germany, monks developed an intensely malty dark beer to help sustain them during prolonged periods of fasting. The beer came to be known as Bock. Later, these same monks brewed an even stronger beer, *Doppelbock,* or "Double-Bock." This new beer was so laden with nutrition that it soon became dubbed "liquid bread" and became the beverage of choice during Lent.

The late English author and renowned beer hunter, **Michael Jackson,** is said to be the top expert and influential voice in the food and drink industries, specifically regarding beer and whiskey and the world's brewing traditions.

His book, *World Guide to Beer,* first published in 1977, is still considered to be the most fundamental book on the subject. The modern theory of "beer style," a term used to differentiate and categorize beers by factors such as color, flavor, strength, ingredients, production method, recipe, history, or origin, began with this book. His books have sold more than three million copies worldwide.

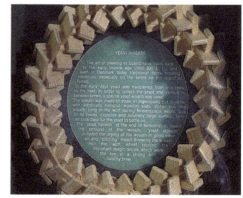
Yeast wreath (courtesy of author)

There are now 60,000+ varieties of beer. One Egyptian pharaoh is reported to have given 16,000 barrels of free beer to his Temple administrator. After the Puritans landed, their production of American hops (Clusters) became so successful that they often shipped them elsewhere.

Thomas Jefferson: "Beer, if drunk in moderation, softens the temper, cheers the spirit, and promotes health."

There are voluminous Wine and Whiskey stories, too, but they would require many additional books.

Plant Scientists — the early explorers and innovators

The amalgamation of plant science and the arts perpetuates the dictum that they enhance each other, giving more joy in their elegant union. The plant scientist Dan Chitwood, as a more contemporary example, has shown how the special grain pattern in the wooden Pernambuco violin bow makes it a most valued asset to professional musicians.

Humboldt

Alexander von Humboldt was an expansive adventurer who traversed practically all of the disciplines of the sciences and arts, and who had an engaging and persuasive persona. His fame in Europe reached a par with Napoleon, yet his engaging friendships with diverse people merits this note.

It was during a reception at the home of Felix Mendelssohn that Humboldt engaged in conversation with Charles Babbage, the futurist computer polymath predictor, as well as his young favorite host, who was just six days short of completing his now well-loved music for *A Midsummer's Night Dream.* Music expanded Humboldt's profound foresight and recognition of nature's diversity. Picture this brave mountain climber reaching Mt. Chimborazo's 19,200 feet without oxygen, proper clothing or a Sherpa guide. He thereafter wrote that high altitude sickness resembled seasickness on land. His diverse interests ranged from geographic and scientific exploration to engineering, ancient and modern languages, painting and the advocacy of human rights. Documenting his life's ideas and adventures required his 5-volume *Kosmos,* which remains highly valued, along with his many other contributions to art and science.

Darwin

Humboldt's meticulous and detailed accomplishments inspired a brilliant Oxford student, Charles Darwin. His adventures began when he journeyed on the HMS Beagle. Darwin could only carry a few books, shelved carefully into the cramped poop-deck space. It took him two and a half years to reach the Pacific Ocean, yet despite his incredible forbearance of an ongoing malady—seasickness—Darwin stated how he abhorred the sea and the ship. Nevertheless, he continued the careful writings of his observations. Inspired by Humboldt's adventurous spirit, he reflected on the "sublime grandeur of the Brazilian Rain Forests."

The innumerable plant collections and meticulous notes about animals he observed on his journey, highlighted by the famous stop at the Galapagos Islands, soon were documented in his controversial 1859 publication *On the Origin of Species*, the original thoughts about speciation and evolution.

His theories were largely supported by few but his confidant, the famous botanist James Hooker. They exchanged over 1400 letters while Darwin worked at home, often despite being chronically ill. Darwin took water cures, meticulous diets and long walks. His illnesses were attributed to hypochondriasis by some, and by others to the South American Chagas disease that is caused by "kissing bug" bites.

Darwin's avoidance of scientific and social meetings probably gave Alfred R. Wallace, his admiring evolutionary competitor, some advantage yet he did not take advantage of it. He did participate in some scientific meetings using modest guidance and reluctant leadership.

Eventually, the importation of tropical plants developed into a hothouse problem for Darwin and many plant scientists, who included…

Richard Spruce

This pioneer traveled extensively through the Amazon and Andes, collecting thousands of specimens for the Kew Gardens. His most notable discovery was the tree in the *Cinchona* genus that produced quinine. Its remarkable curative effect in treating various forms of malaria for untold feverish victims merit attention since resistant forms of *Plasmodium* continue to plague the world. Scientific studies of quinine were first published by Humboldt in the early 18th century. The quinine alkaloid was separated from the powdered bark of *Cinchona* trees and named "quinine" in 1820 by two French doctors.

Ironically, Spruce was plagued with parasitic insects and bouts of malaria. While in the Andes, he suffered a sudden and mysterious paralysis that left him unable to sit upright at his desk. His ongoing observations, however, continued to enhance the study of mosses (http://bryophytes.plant.siu.edu/).

George Washington Carver

George Washington Carver created more than 300 products, greatly improving economic development in the rural South. He promoted crop

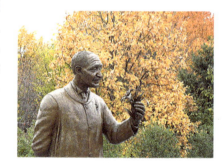

George Washington Carver's statue, Missouri Botanical Garden (courtesy of author)

rotation, growing peanuts, soybeans, and sweet potatoes, while enhancing their market value by inventing hundreds of products to use them. Carver's invention of plant-derived products and his instruction for farmers on how to improve their soil through crop rotation, are his greatest gifts to us. Carver's curiosity, determination, love of nature, and desire to help people were guiding factors in his life.

Norman Borlaug

> "Civilization as it is known today could not have evolved, nor can it survive, without an adequate food supply."
> ~ Norman Borlaug, Ph.D.

Called the father of the Green Revolution, Nobel Peace Prize winner and founder of the World Food Prize Dr. Norman Borlaug has been called "the man who saved more lives than anyone who has ever lived." His research on wheat genetics and other topics continues, inspired by his scientific modesty and diligence. He avoided the "academic butterflies" as a notable pioneer agronomist.

Working with Mexican scientists on problems of wheat improvement, Dr. Borlaug also collaborated with scientists from other parts of the world in adapting the new wheats to new lands. Described as eclectic and pragmatic, Dr. Borlaug was spectacularly successful in finding high-yielding disease-resistant wheat, which he modestly described as "a temporary success in man's war against hunger."

> "Global food production must increase by 70% to feed a population of 9.1 billion people in 2050."
> ~ Food and Agriculture Organization of the United Nations (FAO)

These many successes made Dr. Borlaug a much sought-after adviser to countries whose food production was not keeping pace with their population. The expression "Green Revolution" made Borlaug well-known beyond scientific circles. Despite his popularity and being credited with saving millions of people from starvation, Dr. Borlaug always emphasized that he was "only part of a team."

> "I grew up on the land, on a small farm in NE Iowa. Life was not always easy. I experienced the economic depressions of the 1930s, and from the experience, I felt that families on the land needed help from scientists, and I dedicated my life to science, and especially to food production."
> ~ Norman Borlaug

Paul Talalay

Paul Talalay, MD, Professor of Pharmacology and Molecular Sciences at Johns Hopkins, was an early dedicated proponent of cancer prevention through the intake of specific vegetable diet-derived compounds. He discovered the ability of sulforaphane (from glucoraphanin, a compound produced by cruciferous vegetables) to induce the production of enzymes that help eliminate toxic metabolites from the body. It was proposed that this was one of the mechanisms by which broccoli, especially its sprouts, may help prevent cancer. It also reduces the presence of the gastric bacteria *Helicobacter pylori*, which has been implicated in gastric cancers.

While many dietary elixirs are invariably touted, some astounding and insightful scientists such as Talalay pursued the proposition that plant substances can boost the human body's ability to stave off disease. Specific enzymes convert chemicals to vital substances such as glucosinolates.

These substances are particularly profuse in cruciferous vegetables, especially broccoli sprouts. The abundant sulforaphane enzyme, acting with intestinal bacteria, converts substances into isothiocyanates, specific chemicals that block the development of cancer cells.

Many other scientists are now working diligently to unravel the mysteries of the many interacting factors of plant nutrition.

Jefferson...and Lewis & Clark

> **Cultivators of the earth are the most valuable citizens. They are the most vigorous, the most independent, the most virtuous and they are tied to their country and wedded to its liberty and interests by the most lasting of bonds.**
>
> ~ Thomas Jefferson

President Thomas Jefferson's career reflected his pioneering need to be scientific in all activities, thus rejecting theories having no basis in fact. Long fascinated by the need to explore new lands, he deftly promoted the purchase of the vast Louisiana Territory in 1803, and he turned to Meriwether Lewis, his trusted presidential aide and an Army veteran with experience of the old Northwest. Meriwether mounted a crew of soldiers to accompany him, along with a friend, William Clark, who was designated to map the explorations and specifically to find a water route to the Pacific Ocean.

As a "natural philosopher" (the word 'scientist' did not appear until 1820) of precise standards, Jefferson shared the view that mere speculation of fact had little more use than mere conjectures. He was enthralled with natural phenomena, writing more than two thousand letters of observations and recordings in his Garden Book, replete with notations of soil, crop yields, flower blossoming and even climate changes. He used the term "patient pursuit of facts."

Jefferson's *Farm Book* contains detailed information about farming activities.

In 1795-96, Jefferson wrote short entries outlining the plowing, sowing, planting, and cutting activities, along with concise notes, observations, and calculations about equipment, livestock, workers, plants, crop rotation, and spinning. Jefferson immersed himself in a crash course in botany, zoology, geology, indigenous culture and medicine. He enlisted luminaries such as his own personal physician, Dr. Benjamin Rush, an ardent believer in "bleedings," to help educate him. Subsequently, we find frequent "bleedings," used to treat fevers and diverse illnesses and wounds, embedded in his logs.

The Corps of Discovery consisted of a select group of U.S. Army volunteers under the command of Captain Lewis and Second Lieutenant William Clark. It took over two years to complete this mission, replete with many new discoveries.

Cacti were not the only hazard; their moccasins were worn through within a month's time.

There was one case of appendicitis, innumerable bouts of diarrhea, profound fatigue and many lacerations. Moving into the Great Plains, the expedition began to see animals unknown in the East: coyotes, antelope, mule deer, and others. On one particular day, all the men were employed drowning a prairie dog out of its hole for shipment back to Jefferson. In all, the captains would describe in their journals 178 plants and 122 animals that previously had not been recorded for science.

December 17
Clark notes a temperature of 45 degrees below zero – "colder," John Ordway adds, "than I ever knew it be in the States." A week later, on Christmas Eve, Fort Mandan was deemed complete and the expedition has moved in for the winter.

February 11
Sacagawea gives birth to a baby boy, Jean Baptiste. Lewis assisted with the difficult delivery by using a folk remedy—a rattlesnake's rattle, crushed and dissolved in water. Lewis and Clark dispatched the big keelboat and roughly a dozen men back downriver, collecting maps, reports, Indian artifacts, and boxes of scientific specimens for Jefferson (including Indian corn, animal skins and skeletons, mineral samples, and five live animals including the prairie dog).

Crop Biotechnology Today (with a nod to Jefferson)

> *Some argue that now isn't the time to push the green agenda—that all efforts should be on preventing a serious recession. That is a false choice. It fails to recognize that climate change and our carbon reliance is part of the problem. High fuel prices and food shortages due to poor crop yields compound today's financial difficulties.*
>
> ~ Lucy Powell, Labour MP, 2008

GMOs

Should plants, animals or microorganisms be genetically modified?

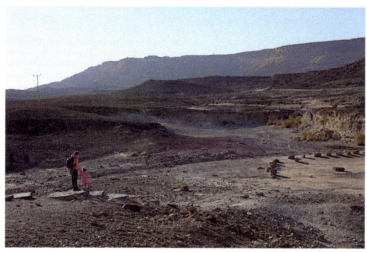

Negev Desert (courtesy of author)

Proponents point to astounding successes in the Philippines. Since the adoption of biotechniques to produce more corn, there has been a 22% increase in yield, a 37% decrease in pesticide use, and a 68% increase in net profits for some of the poorest farmers in the world. GM seeds improve plant durability by making them disease resistant; they will raise drought tolerance, increasing crop yield, lowering costs and improving nutritional value. The demand for high-yield pest-resistant crops remains constant due to the need to feed the world's growing population on a decreasing acreage of arable land. Gains of over $100 billion dollars in sixteen years have allegedly been demonstrated from lower pest and weed losses using genetic methods.

Scientists have been able to genetically modify cassava by incorporating Vitamin A, preventing blindness in over 250,000 children.

EuropaBio, the European Association for Bioindustries, promotes the innovative and dynamic European industry and is committed to improve quality of life; to prevent, diagnose, treat and cure diseases; to improve the quality and quantity of food and feedstuffs; and to move towards a bio-based and zero-waste economy.

In the U.S. the FDA regulates the safety of food for humans and animals, including foods from genetically modified (GM) plants. The FDA requires developers to conduct safety trials before marketing their products.

Conserving biodiversity and perpetuating the prior indigenous co-partnership knowledge seem destined to amplify the future beneficial pharmacopoeias. The many secondary gains with the ubiquitous plant kingdom will preserve food supplies and lead to needed cures of refractory illnesses.

A new approach follows Nature's schemes—why not?

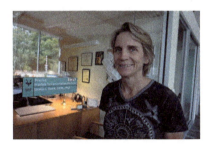

Dr. Sharon Deem (courtesy of author)

Manure into methane

Mike McCloskey, who runs one of the largest U.S. dairy operations, has produced an industrial model that evokes praise for its conservation and yields of milk as well as methane-based fuel. It converts cow manure into methane to power dairies and then turns it into compressed natural gas to fuel a fleet of 42 CNG-powered tractor trailers. This one critical innovation eliminates the equivalent of 12 million miles of fossil fuel emissions annually. The goal is to eventually run the world's first dairy farm with a carbon neutral footprint (fortune.com, 2/1/16). Some fuel powers the farm; other conversions produce compressed natural gas. Residuals are used as a non-toxic fertilizer, to produce crops that feed the cattle.

Drones

Grape vineyards are now monitored by drones to better define effects of drought and temperature alterations. Multispectral imagery detects vegetation abnormalities, preventing crop disasters. These drones may identify areas of pests, disease, and weeds; collect tissue for fertility and disease tests; collect soil samples for soil, fertility, pH and pest issues; inspect root structure for signs of compaction, depth, disease, and pests; measure erosion channel width and depth; and note machine issues and defects.

Lower-tech tech—banking the seeds we need

> " From a small seed a mighty trunk may grow. "
>
> ~ Aeschylus

> " The lucrative aspects of importing seeds, bulbs and some plants generated bartering for commerce while improving botanical studies. "
>
> ~ Daniel Chamovitz

The Norwegian Svalbard Bank stores over 1 million specimens, each available should there be a world catastrophe.

Seeds have long been considered a potent sexual stimulant, and have been sought for millennia and reaped huge fortunes. Think about the vastness of the desert and its potential source of nourishment with supplemental minerals to feed us for years. Large areas are irrigated for agriculture and many Israeli communities have been established there. Meanwhile, plants continue their silent filtering and shading functions that increase the supplies of farmed fish and safe and plentiful foods.

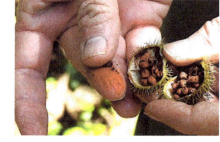

Achiote seeds used to create lipstick (courtesy of author)

Trees & Leaves & Us

We have decimated trees, yet our health and earth depend on their survival. Trees combat climate change: they absorb CO_2 by removing and storing the carbon while releasing oxygen back into the air. A perfect symphonic theme. The Moreton Bay Fig tree in San Diego is believed to be the largest *Ficus macrophylla* in the United States. There are some parasitic trees, such as the "strangler fig," that may harm, yet strengthen, the host tree during storms by insulating and compressing its branches. The terebinth tree has been known to live over one thousand years, has a width greater than 20 feet, and merited multiple mentions in the Bible.

A harmonious display of interacting tall trees provides benefits for cities and towns as a standard mission. Trees also provide us with many musical instruments, often formed from the treasured wood of rare jungle species. Examples include the Amazonian Pernambuco bows, the Stradivari violins, the woodwinds and so many other assets to our joy in living. Clothing, too, has been fashioned from plant fibers and bark.

Trees also clean the air by absorbing odor and pollutant gases (nitrogen oxides, ammonia, sulfur dioxide and ozone) and filter particulates out of the air by trapping them in their leaves and bark.

Average temperatures in Los Angeles have risen six degrees Fahrenheit in the last 50 years as tree coverage in the city has declined and the number of heat-absorbing roads and buildings has increased. Trees cool the city up to ten degrees Fahrenheit, by shading our homes and streets, breaking up urban "heat islands," and releasing water vapor into the air through their leaves.

Tree bark growth continues as does its century-old scaffolding, dwarfing and humbling us, yet providing our lumber products for extensive building of furniture, homes and water conveyances.

We are aware that leaves' shapes, with their multi-colored patterns, appear universally, yet the diverse underlying anatomical and physiological features are seldom apparent. Recent science has indicated that leaf size depends on climatic and altitude conditions.

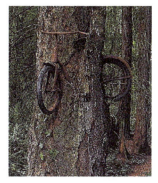

Bike swallowed by tree (Jason Wilson, photographer, https://www.flickr.com/photos/hive/4075884)

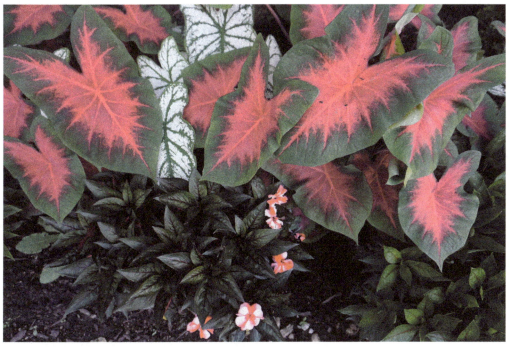

Caladium leaves (courtesy of author)

Asters (courtesy of author)

The precise screening of the leaves that are shipped daily to the Missouri Botanical Garden herbarium from throughout the world requires unique skills.

Genes function as controllers of leaf shapes and their precise patterns. The green pigment known as chlorophyll diminishes with the onset of cool weather in autumn. When abundant in the leaf's pigment cells during the growing season, the green color dominates and masks out the colors of any other pigments that may be present. Inside the leaf, a chloroplast organelle loses its color as the underlying red, yellow and orange colors dominate.

Fall foliage tourists often travel as "Leaf Peepers," following all weather reports, and experience their own visceral responses that are accentuated by nature's chromatic paint brush.

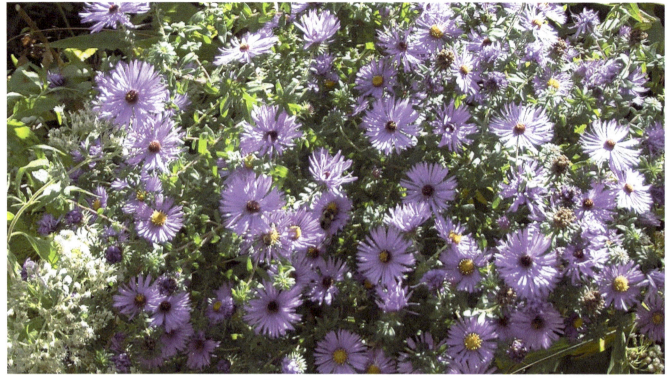

Ronald Liesner, curatorial assistant at Missouri Botanical Garden (courtesy of author)

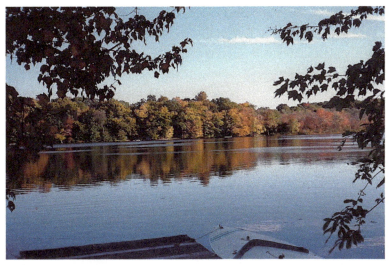

Linsley Lake, North Branford, Connecticut (courtesy of author)

This autumn scene shows a heavily studied 15,000-year-old glacial lake, where several Yale University Ph.D. students conducted research for their doctoral dissertations. All their studies related to the changing flora and chemistry of the lake as influenced by human habitations.

Pollinators & Colony Collapse

Pollination is the process by which pollen is transferred to the female reproductive organs of plants and is followed by fertilization. Multiple bee pollinators respond to olfactory and nectar signals within distinct plant species. Insects, birds, bats, and the wind transport pollen among flowering plants, thereby enabling diverse chemical profiles. Only lately have scientists defined microscopic pollen grain reproductive activities within the stems.

> **A bee is an exquisite chemist.**
> ~ Royal Beekeeper to Charles II

In the six years leading up to 2013, more than 10 million

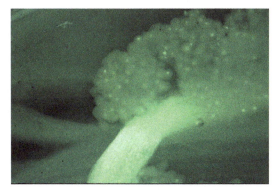

Pollen inside a leaf stem (courtesy of author, taken in the lab of Dr. Peter Bernhardt)

beehives were lost—twice the normal rate, and often to Colony Collapse Disorder (CCD). A profound disruption of food supplies may owe to this 'bee collapse,' which is intimately related to contamination with fertilizers—though many scientists cite additional causes.

The economic value of honey bees' pollination of plants globally was estimated to be close to $200 billion in 2005. Shortages of bees in the U.S. have increased the cost to farmers, who must now rent bees for pollination services. CCD remains an unsolved problem, though nicotinamide specifically has been implicated as a cause. Lobbying to exclude fertilizers known to damage bee terrain has been unsuccessful, as agricultural corporations vigorously deny the toxicity of their products as their wealth continues to grow.

Other important pollinators such as bats, birds, butterflies and even crickets also seem vulnerable to toxic agents employed routinely for weed control. Bats serve a vital role in protecting plants (even if they also carry coronaviruses), as they devour nematode larvae—which is why the recent proliferation of the fungal white-nose syndrome has the potential to seriously threaten our food supplies.

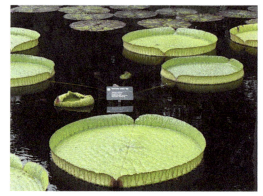

Lily pads at the Missouri Botanical Garden (courtesy of author)

Short Notes — stem cells, weeds, marijuana (*the* weed) & ginger

Plant and human stem cells are multipotent cells that can differentiate into a variety of cell types, which may serve as an internal repair system that replicates as needed to replace damaged tissue. These special embryonic cells are currently being studied as to how they might lead to better control of viruses, parasites, and other invaders of food crops including wheat, cassava and other essential foods. The Yale Stem Cell Center has defined the role of stem cells in limiting brain metastases, renewing surviving beta cells in type 1 childhood diabetes, and other potential functions.

> "Embryonic stem cell research will prolong life, improve life and give hope for life to millions of people"
>
> ~ Jim Ramstad, former Minnesota congressman

Publications of Dr. Yung-Chi Cheng of Yale University have led to pathways for treatment of metastatic carcinomas. In addition, plant tissue stem cell research promises great advancements. Recent leaf spectro-scanning permits almost minuscule leaf examinations using cell phones and other available devices and software.

An astounding new research tool, the Titan Krios cryo-electron microscope, has now given us crystallized 3D images smaller than an atom. The application to plant science research is eagerly awaited.

Some chemicals manufactured to control weeds have proven to be toxic and potentially threatening to human health. A few have been shown to be safe. Kudzu was introduced in North America in 1876 in the southeastern U.S. to prevent soil erosion. But kudzu spread quickly and soon overtook farms and buildings, leading some to call it "the vine that ate the South." Its root has been used to treat alcoholism and as a mild pain killer, despite the worry that it might be an addictive opioid. Health providers in China sometimes give intravenous puerarin, a chemical in kudzu, to dissolve blood clots in the treatment of stroke.

> "What is a weed? A plant whose virtues have not yet been discovered."
>
> ~ Ralph Waldo Emerson

The long-famous marijuana plant, *Cannabis sativa,* is a type of hemp. Cannabinoids continue to vie for legal status, since they have been shown to be useful in reducing pain, especially in cancer patients. Others stress that this "weed" has some addicting properties despite its soothing pain relief action. Pain relief remains the mantra while many nations have approved over-the-counter availability.

The centuries-old poppy plant extract, morphine, remains consistently popular as an opioid of choice.

As early as 500 BC, ginger was used as a medicine and for flavoring food in ancient China and India. In the western hemisphere, ginger was used to spice drinks. During the Victorian era, it was used to brew an alcoholic beverage known as "ginger beer." Throughout history, ginger beer has been used as a remedy for all sorts of maladies and illnesses. Ginger is considered an anti-inflammatory, digestive aid, and an aid for pregnant women suffering from morning sickness. This is yet another example of how many plants are both food and medicine.

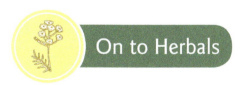

On to Herbals

We are currently discovering the latent treasures of Chinese herbals that have been used by Asian physicians for centuries. Some have anti-cancer properties that eliminate metastases and others are revealing the occult chemistries of many tumors. We have yet to explore these latent Chinese herbal benefits in full but they are very promising. Anti-cancer drugs for metastatic disease are now advancing to the final stage of human research trials.

Every herbal has a story. The practice of ingesting bilberry to improve night vision predates its use by Royal Air Force (RAF) pilots in World War II. The bilberry increases capillary flow by dilating vessels and preventing leakage. It is useful for treating varicosities and spider skin lesions and has been shown to prevent cataracts and myopia. It also is a major ingredient in some jams and jellies. Bilberry fruit contains plant pigments that have excellent antioxidant properties. They scavenge damaging particles in the body known as free radicals, and thereby help to prevent or reverse damage to cells. Antioxidants have been shown to help prevent a number of long-term illnesses, such as heart disease and cancer. Bilberry may also be useful in treating macular degeneration. This fruit also contains Vitamin C, another antioxidant.

Sniffing lavender has been said to relieve stress. Considered the most popular of the nostalgic organic fragrances, lavender can allegedly bring back memories of happy childhood times, delivering up sweet sensations and drowsy summer fields. But lavender is more than just a pleasing floral scent. One of the most powerful medicines in the plant world, it provided both physical and emotional relief for Egyptians and others in the ancient world.

Close to one third of modern prescription medicines contain a plant-derived ingredient, and chemicals from plants have contributed to the production of many useful synthetic compounds and pharmaceuticals.

What Are Your Symptoms? — consider plants (& pesticides)

Toxins

TOXIC HAZARD

Symptoms become subtle diagnostic crystal-ball challenges for clinicians who properly assess modern travelers, expatriates and herbal enthusiasts for latent exposures.

The recent use of the common herbicide glyphosate containing 2,4-D in an attempt to control milkweed growth has now reduced the population of monarch butterflies by 30%, as these species depend on milkweed for survival. This chemical may also induce human cancer and thyroid problems. Roundup and other glyphosate-based herbicides are now extensively applied to genetically modified corn, soy and cotton in 34 states.

Analgesic and heart preparations containing highly toxic aconite alkaloids have produced paralysis, heart irregularity and death. Other root concoctions such as Konzo contain the cyanogens in un-boiled cassava roots. Bonesetter's herbs, "Zheng Gu Shui" and "Tieh Ta Yao Gin," which are used to reduce post-traumatic pain and swelling, each contain myrrh, which is a putative dermatitis allergen.

The "medicinal" use of licorice (glycyrrhetinic acid) may induce essential hypertension. Drinking or smoking the resin of boiled jimson weed seeds produces severe anticholinergic toxicity in the brain, and is similar to the toxicity of herbal Paraguay tea—which induces prominent bizarre mental changes (colloquially described as "mad as a hatter"), and the bowel and bladder lose their tone and the heart beats abnormally.

Many plants produce alkaloids. Liver specialists are wary of at least nine pyrrolizidines that are found in some prepared foods and that can cause veno-occlusive liver disease. Foxglove (digitalis), while often mistaken for a bush herbal, is often used to make tea, and might produce a digitalis excess. Other non–food toxins extracted from plants are found in factory and auto repair shops, their exposure awaiting potential associations with serious liver disease. It has been suggested that some factory fumes might cause liver necrosis in beer drinkers or produce visual loss, pancreatitis, or the urinary oxalate crystals in kidney stones.

Other toxins found in Asian herbals include lead or arsenic, which might be found on the metal utensils or the brewing pottery or in the tea leaves. These agents can also include ethylene glycol, methanol, ethanol, propylene glycol, and carbon tetrachloride.

Some beads for children may still be made of seeds despite being the occasional cause of contact skin eruptions. Chewing a specific necklace seed may lead to severe abdominal pain, diarrhea, dehydration, and oliguria. One must immediately arrange admission to a pediatric ICU while you dial the National Hotline Number: 1-800-222-1222 or 800-CDC-INFO to identify the problem.

The castor bean is processed to make castor oil, but the mash waste contains ricin. Toxic poisoning by inhalation or ingestion promptly produces severe symptoms of organ failure. A lethal dose is as small as a grain of salt. Rapid emergency care is vital to survival.

The profound proliferation of current nutritional and food supplements, despite the potential toxicity with heavy metals and carcinogens, now further challenges clinicians. The advertised herbal "benefits" of body slimming, increased sexual prowess, ageless facial renewal, astounding energy enhancement and cures for many chronic illnesses invite subtle diagnostic dilemmas. Herbal uses are often withheld by patients, producing management puzzles, especially when occult drug interactions occur. The onset of blood loss, abrupt renal-liver failure, menstrual irregularities and confusing states all may result from latent herbal usage.

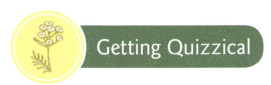

Getting Quizzical

Before Captain Cook was killed by Polynesian natives, what two plant products did he insist his sailors ingest to save them from an illness producing strange mouth and extremity hair conditions?[1]

Sailors suffered from scurvy caused by a lack of Vitamin C. Patients may display characteristic curly hair on the arms and legs and have decaying teeth and gums.

---

[1] cabbage, citrus fruits

16th-century monks are said to have chewed on certain berries to repress their sexual desires. Can you name that berry?[2]

And can you name three other aphrodisiac herbals?[3]

A woman with borderline congestive heart failure was admitted to the hospital and found to have toxic digitalis levels. At the same time, the laboratory reported that her INR and prothrombin levels were excessively high. She denied taking extra heart pills. Questioning the contents of her bulging medicine cabinet revealed that she believed in the pharmaceutical efficacy of herbals.

Suspecting only occupational sources for heavy metal poisoning may overlook the contamination of many health food products as well as the toxic potential of NSAIDs (anti-inflammatory drugs), steroids and microorganisms.

Correlation of Signs & Symptoms — a comprehensive Plants R Cures chart

Correlation of Plants & Symptoms

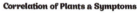
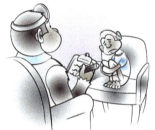

Once again, recall Soma Weiss' sage admonition:

 A diagnosis is easy, as long as you think of it.

Future Potentials

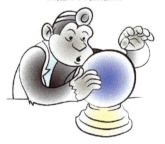

The author's differential diagnostic sections below are readily identified and compartmentalized within their viral, parasitic, bacterial, fungal and plant domains.

Hopefully, the index chart will enlighten or aid in reinforcement of prior knowledge.

---

[2] chase tree

[3] gingko biloba, ginseng, yohimbe

VIRUSES	HELMINTHS	PROTOZOA	BACTERIA	OTHERS	** PLANT TREATMENTS **
		ABDOMINAL DISTENTION			
	STRONGYLOIDIASIS TRICHURIASIS	AMEBIASIS, GIARDIASIS, KALA AZAR	BOTULISM, PIG BEL, RICKETTSIOSES (TYPHUS & R.M.T.S. FEVER)		PAPAYA, PEPPERMINT LEAVES; GINGER ROOT, FENNEL SEEDS, SAW PALMETTO BERRIES
		ABDOMINAL TENDERNESS WITH OR WITHOUT MASS			
DENGUE EBOLA VIRUS HEMORR. WITH RENAL SYNDROME RIFT VALLEY FEVER	ANGIOSTRONGYLIASIS ANISAKIASIS ENTEROBIASIS OPISTHORCHIASIS SCHISTOSOMIASIS STRONGYLOIDIASIS TAENIASIS TRICHURIASIS	AMEBOMA, AMEBIC COLITIS, BALANTIDIASIS F. MALARIA TOXOPLASMOSIS	ANTHRAX CAMPYLOBACTER LYME DISEASE SALMONELLOSIS SHIGELLOSIS RICKETTSIOSES TERTIARY SYPHILIS YERSINIOSIS	PANCREATITIS TRACHOMATIS SPIDER & TICK BITE-INDUCED SYNDROME	PAPAYA, PEPPERMINT LEAVES
		ANEMIA – HEMORRHAGE, ACUTE & CHRONIC			
AIDS, CHIKUNGUNYA FEVER	DIPHYLLOBOTHRIASIS FASCIOLOPSIS BUSKI	AMEBIASIS	BARTONELLOSIS (CARRION'S DIS) HISTOPLASMOSIS	MYIASIS, VIPERINE SNAKE BITE	GENTIAN FOR DISABILITY, GINSENG
EBOLA, MARBURG	HOOKWORM	BABESIOSIS BALANTIDIASIS	LEPTOSPIROSIS RELAPSING FEVER		NETTLE, YARROW
RIFT VALLEY & OTHER HEMORRHAGIC FEVERS	SCHISTOSOMIASIS TRICHURIASIS		SHIGELLOSIS TUBERCULOSIS TYPHOID FEVER, TYPHUS	QUININE SENSITIVITY	SAW PALMETTO, NETTLE
		ANURIA & OLIGURIA			
AIDS EB VIRUS HEMORRHAGIC FEVERS WITH RENAL SYNDROME, YELLOW FEVERS	LOIASIS SCHISTOSOMIASIS (HEMATOBIUM)	BABESIA BOVIS F. MALARIA	CHOLERA, LEPTOSPIROSIS (R.M.T.S. FEVER & TYPHUS), SHIGELLOSIS, TULAREMIA	GIANT DESERT CENTIPEDE BITE	
		ASCITES			
DECOMPENSATED HEPATITIS (ASSOC. VENO-OCCLUSIVE HEPATOCELLULAR CA)	CAPILLARIASIS CLONORCHIASIS		ANTHRAX TUBERCULOSIS	GORDOLOBO/ YERBA TEA INGESTION (RENO-OCCLUSIVE LIVER TOXICITY)	

VIRUSES	HELMINTHS	PROTOZOA	BACTERIA	OTHERS	** PLANT TREATMENTS **
CARDIOMYOPATHY					
AIDS, COXSACKIE, MARBURG DISEASE, YELLOW FEVER	DIROFILARIA, LOIASIS (ENDOMYOCARDIAL FIBROSIS), TRICHINOSIS	AMEBIASIS, F. MALARIA, TOXOPLASMOSIS, TRYPANOSOMIASIS	DIPHTHERIA TOXIN, BRUCELLOSIS, LYME DISEASE, Q FEVER	ASPERGILLOSIS, COCAINE TOXICITY, CHILAMYDIA, ORNITHOSIS, PSITTICOSIS, STONEFISH INJURY	PRIMROSE, GENTIAN & GINGER
CLUBBING					
	PARAGONIMIASIS SCHISTOSOMIASIS (INTEST & PULMON INVOLVEMENT)	AMEBIASIS		VARIOUS MALIGNANCIES	
COMA					
AIDS ARBOVIRUS	ANGIOSTRONGYLIASIS	ACANTHAMOEBIASIS (NAEGLERIA)	LEPTOSPIROSIS MENINGOCOCCEMIA	CRYPTOCOCCOSIS INGESTED POISONING	
ENCEPHALITIDES	CAPILLARIASIS		R.M.T.S. FEVER TYPHOID FEVER	AKEE, CASSAVA, SHELLFISH	
EBOLA, LASSA FEVER, RIFT VALLEY FEVER, VIRAL HEPATITIS, MEASLES, RABIES	CESTODIASES (T. SOLIUM)	F. MALARIA TRYPANOSOMIASIS	TYPHUS, LEPTOSPIROSIS	MT. ALTITUDE SYN VIPERINE SNAKE & SPIDER	
VALLEY FEVER, VIRAL HEPATITIS, MEASLES, RABIES (RARE)	PARAGONIMIASIS SCHISTOSOMIASIS (RARE), TRICHINOSIS			BITES (NEUROTOXIC ENVENOMING)	HALLUCINOGENICS; KAVA; NUTMEG
CONFUSIONAL STATE					JIMSON WEED; YOHIMBE
ARBOVIRUS ENCEPHALITIDES DENGUE	CYSTICEROSIS EHCINOCOCCOSIS (E. GRANULOSUS)	AMEBIASIS, F. MALARIA, TOXOPLASMOSIS, TRYPANOSOMIASIS	ANTHRAX, CAT SCRATCH, LISTERIOSIS, LYME DISEASE	BROMIDISM ERGOTISM FUNGAL MENINGITIS MT. ALTITUDE SYN	CAUTIOUS WITH STIMULANTS: SENNA, CASCARA, BRAN, CINNAMON, GARLIC, FENNEL SEED, FLAXSEED, RHUBARB ROOT
LASSA FEVER, RABIES			NEISSERIA MENINGITIDIS NEUROSYPHILIS PLAGUE (Y. PESTIS) RICKETTSIOSIS	INSECTICIDES	

VIRUSES	HELMINTHS	PROTOZOA	BACTERIA	OTHERS	** PLANT TREATMENTS **
		CONSTIPATION & INTESTINAL OBSTRUCTION			
DENGUE EARLY POLIO	ANISAKIASIS ASCARIASIS DIPHYLLOBOTHRIASIS FASCIOLOPSIASIS (MUCOID STOOLS) SCHISTOSOMIASIS	AMEBIASIS, CHAGAS	BOTULISM, TYPHOID FEVER	HISTOPLASMOSIS	SENNA; FLAXSEED; RHUBAB
		COUGH & RESPIRATORY SYMPTOMS			
LASSA FEVER, MEASLES	ASCARIASIS (LOEFFLER'S SYNDROME)	AMEBIASIS CHAGAS (ESOPH. REGURGITATION)	ANTHRAX BRANHAMELLA	ACTINOMYCOSIS ASPERGILLOSIS	MENTHOL, FENNEL, HYSSOP, GINKGO BILOBA, LICORICE, MULLEIN, SARSAPARILLA
POLIO	ECHINOCOCCOSIS HOOKWORM	CRYPTOSPORIDIOSIS	CATARRHALIS LEGIONNAIRES	BLASTOMYCOSIS CANDIDIASIS	
RABIES	PARAGONIMIASIS	PNEUMOCYSTOSIS	PLAGUE	CHLAMYDIAE	MYRRH, EVENING PRIMROSE, CAPSAICIN OINTMENT, ALOE, WITCH HAZEL LEMON BALM, MALLOW, LICORICE, SARSAPARILLA, TEA TREE OIL, NETTLE
		TOXOPLASMOSIS VISCERAL LEISHMANIASIS	RICKETTSIOSES TYPHOID FEVER TUBERCULOSIS TULAREMIA	COCCICIODIDO, HISTOPLASMOSIS, MT. ALTITUDE SYNDROMES, NEUROTOXIC EN-VENOMING, SPOROTRICHOSIS	HAWTHORN
		CUTANEOUS			
AIDS (KAPOSI), DENGUE, MEASLES, PAPILLOMA VIRUSES, TICK-BORNE HEMORRHAGIC FEVERS, YELLOW FEVER	CREEPING ERUPTION (ANCYLOSTOMA), DRACUNCULIASIS, ECHINOCOCCOSIS, ENTEROBIASIS, LOIASIS, ONCHOCERCIASIS, PARAGONIMIASIS, SCHISTOSOMIASIS, KATAYAMA FEVER, SWIMMER'S ITCH, STRONGYLOIDIASIS, TOXOCARIASIS, TRICIHINOSIS	LEISHMANIASIS TOXOPLASMOSIS TRYPANOSOMIASIS	ANTHRAX, ASPERGILLOSIS, CAT SCRATCH DISEASE, LEPROSY, LYME DISEASE, MENINGOCOCCEMIA, ALL RICKETTSIOSES, SYPHILIS, TULAREMIA, TYPHOID FEVER, TYPHUS, TOXIC SHOCK SYN. VIBRIOSIS: PARAHAEMOLYTICUS, VULNIFICUS	BLASTOMYCOSIS, COCCIDIOSIS, LEPROSY, MYCETOMA, SCABIES (NOCTURNAL PRURITUS), SPOROTRICHOSIS, VENOMOUS BITES & STINGS, YAWS	HERPES SIMPLEX: LEMON GEL, SIBERIAN GINSENG. ANTIFUNGAL: TEA TREE OIL. SUNBURN: ALOE GEL, CHAMOMILE, BLACK CURRANT OIL, EVENING PRIMROSE OIL

VIRUSES	HELMINTHS	PROTOZOA	BACTERIA	OTHERS	** PLANT TREATMENTS **
		DIARRHEA			
AIDS, EBOLA DISEASE	CAPILLARIASIS PARAGONIMIASIS	AMEBIASIS BALANTIDIASIS	B. CEREUS	CIGUATOXIN COCCIDIOSIS	RASPBERRY, BILBERRY, WITCH HAZEL
		CRYPTOSPORIDOSIS	C. PERFRINGENS	FISH STINGS	
MARBURG, MEASLES	FASCIOLOPSIASIS SCHISTOSOMIASIS	GIARDIASIS	(PIG BEL), E. COLI		
	STRONGYLOIDIASIS TRICHINOSIS TRICHURIASIS	LEISHMANIASIS EARLY F. MALARIA TOXOPLASMOSIS	ENTEROTOX, ENTEROHEMORR, LISTERIOSIS, SALMONELLOSIS, SHIGELLOSIS, TUBERCULOSIS (ILEOCECAL), YERSINIA, ENTERO-COLITICA	INGESTED POISONINGS e.g. MUSHROOM SCOMBROTOXIN ENVENOMATIONS	
		FEVER			
AIDS, ARBOVIRUSES, LASSA FEVER, ETC., DENGUE	FASCIOLIASIS, SCHISTOSOMIASIS (EARLY), TOXOCARIASIS	LEISHMANIASIS (VISCERAL & MUCOCUTANEOUS) MALARIA	ANTHRAX BARTONELLOSIS BRUCELLOSIS CAMPYLOBACTER LEGIONNAIRES	DRUG REACTIONS & VARIOUS FOOD TOXINS e.g. CIGUATERA, MUSHROOM	YARROW (ACHILLEA MILLEFOLIUM)
RABIES, VIRAL ENCEPHALITIS	TRICHINOSIS	PRIMARY AMEBIC MENINGOENCEPHALITIS	LEPTOSPIROSIS, LYME DISEASE	INGESTED POISONS	
YELLOW FEVER (FAGET'S SIGN)		TOXOPLASMOSIS TRYPANOSOMIASIS	LISTERIOSIS, NOCARDIOSIS, PLAGUE, RELAPSING FEVER, RICKETTSIOSES, SHIGELLOSIS, SECONDARY SYPHILIS, TUBERCULOSIS, TYPHOID, TYPHUS	FUNGAL DISEASES	
		HEMATURIA & HEMOGLOBINURIA			
VIRAL HEMORRHAGIC FEVER WITH RENAL SYNDROME, YELLOW FEVER	SCHISTOSOMIASIS (HAEMATOMA) FILARIASIS	FALCIPARUM, MALARIA	LEPTOSPIROSIS, SYPHILIS, TYPHUS	VIPERINE & SNAKE BITES, G6PD DEFICIENCY. INGESTED POISONS: FAVISM, QUININE	
		HEPATOMEGALY			
DENGUE EB VIRUS VIRAL HEPATITIS YELLOW FEVER	ECHINOCOCCOSIS FASCIOLIASIS SCHISTOSOMIASIS (ESP. KATAYAMA FEVER)	AMEBIASIS, BABESIOSIS, MALARIA, TRYPANOSOMIASIS	BACTEROIDES BRUCELLOSIS LEPTOSPIROSIS LISTERIOSIS	CHLAMYDIAE PSITTACOSIS C. TRACHOMATIS	

VIRUSES	HELMINTHS	PROTOZOA	BACTERIA	OTHERS	** PLANT TREATMENTS **
	TOXOCARIASIS	(CHAGAS) VISCERAL LEISHMANIASIS TOXOPLASMOSIS	LYME DISEASE, RELAPSING FEVER, RICKETTSIOSES, TULAREMIA, TYPHOID FEVER	DISSEMINATED HISTOPLASMOSIS, RELAPSING FEVER	

JAUNDICE

VIRUSES	HELMINTHS	PROTOZOA	BACTERIA	OTHERS	** PLANT TREATMENTS **
				INGESTED POISONS	

LABORATORY CLUES

VIRUSES	HELMINTHS	PROTOZOA	BACTERIA	OTHERS	** PLANT TREATMENTS **
	ANGIOSTRONGYLUS	EOSINOPHILIA		ASPERGILLOSIS	
	ASCARIASIS	LEPROSY	SCABIES		
	CAPILLARIASIS, CESTODIASIS, CLONORCHIASIS, DRACUNCULIASIS, ECHINOCOCCOSIS, FASCIOLIASIS, FILARIASIS, HOOKWORM, LOIASIS, ONCHOCERCIASIS, PARAGONIMIASIS, SCHISTOSOMIASIS, STRONGYLOIDIASIS, TOXOCARIASIS, TRICHINOSIS, TRICHURIASUS			COCCIDIODOMYCOSIS EOSINOPHILIA-MYALGIA SYNDROME (L-TRYPTOPHAN INGESTION) TROPICAL EOSINOPHILIA	

INCREASED IMMUNOGLOBULINEMIA

VIRUSES	HELMINTHS	PROTOZOA	BACTERIA	OTHERS	** PLANT TREATMENTS **
	THRICHINOSIS			MYELOMA	
		LEUKEMOID			
	TRICHINOSIS				
		MONOCYTOSIS			
EB VIRUS; AIDS					
		NEUTROPENIA			
				MARROW DEPRESSIONS	
		PROTEINURIA			
				RENAL FAILURE, MYELOMAS	
		THROMBOCYTOPENIA			

VIRUSES	HELMINTHS	PROTOZOA	BACTERIA	OTHERS	** PLANT TREATMENTS **
		LYMPHADENOPATHY			
AIDS		SYPHILIS		LYMPHOMAS; NEOPLASIA	
		NEURASTHENIA & PSEUDOPSYCHOGENIC			
		OCULAR			
		VASCULAR			FOR VASCULAR PROBLEMS
		VULNERABLE WHEN IMMUNOCOMPROMISED STATE			
					HORSE CHESTNUT (FOR PHLEBITIS, VARICOSITIES, HEMORRHOIDS- TIGHTENS VESSELS)
		VULNERABLE WHEN SPLENECTOMY STATE			
		BABIOSIS			
		LYMPHOMAS			
AIDS CMV		AMEBIASIS GIARDIASIS		NEOPLASIA; HYPERTHYROIDISM	
		ADRENAL INSUFFICIENCY			
				SEPSIS	
		ANGIOEDEMA			
AIDS	TRICHINOSIS				
		BACK PAIN			FEVERFEW, GINGER, NETTLE, SARSAPARILLLA, TURMERIC, YUCCA, CAPSAICIN, GINGER
AIDS DENGUE FEVER		MALARIA	BRUCELLOCISIS	TRAUMA	
		BONE PAIN & LESIONS			
				NEOPLASIA	

VIRUSES	HELMINTHS	PROTOZOA	BACTERIA	OTHERS	** PLANT TREATMENTS **
		BREAST LESIONS			MULLEIN, NETTLE, WILD YAM. HYPOGLYCEMIC HERBS: GINSENG, KOREAN GINSENG
AIDS	NEMATODE INTRUSIONS				
		DIABETIC STATES			
		EPIDIDYMO ORCHITIS			
MUMPS					
		EPISTAXIS			
		AMEBIASIS			
		ERYTHEMA NODOSUM			
		FETID BREATH & OLFACTORY AIDS			
			TYPHOID	RENAL & HEPATIC FAILURE; KETOSIS	
		GASTRECTOMY STATUS – VULNERABLILITES:			
		HYDROPHOBIA			
			TETANUS		
		NAILS – SPLINTER HEMORRHAGES			
	TRICHINOSIS		VARIOUS INFECTIVE ENDOCARDITIS		
		NEOPLASIA: POTENTIAL ASSOCIATIONS			
		PANCREATITIS			
	NEMATODE INTRUSIONS			ASSOC. COMMON DUCT OBSTRUCTIONS	
		PERICARDITIS & EFFUSION			
AIDS CMV	TRICHINOSIS	AMEBIASIS		POST-CATHETERIZATION	
		PELVIC PAIN, CHRONIC (P.I.D.)			
AIDS					

VIRUSES	HELMINTHS	PROTOZOA	BACTERIA	OTHERS	** PLANT TREATMENTS **
		PLEURAL EFFUSION			
AIDS CMV		AMEBIASIS		NEOPLASIA	
		POLYARTHRALGIA			
AIDS	TRICHINOSIS	LYME		METAL POISONING	
		RECTAL DISORDERS			
		PROLAPSE		HEMORRHOIDS	
	AMEBIASIS				
		PROCTITIS			
LYMPHOGRANULOMA	TRICHURIASIS; ASCARIASIS	AMEBIASIS		LOCAL TRAUMA	
	PINWORMS; TRICHURIASIS			HEMORRHOIDS	
		RECTAL ULCERS			
AIDS; LYMPHOGRANULOMA		AMEBIASIS	SYPHILIS	LOCAL TRAUMA	
		SALT CRAVING			
		FISH TAPEWORM		ADDISONIAN STATUS	
		SPLENOMEGALY			
		LYME DISEASE		TRAUMA	
		TASTE ABERRATIONS			
				CIGUATERA	
		TRISMUS			
			TETANUS	DENTAL INFECTION	
		TRANSFUSIONS – TRANSMISSIONPOTENTIALS			
CMV AIDS; VIRAL HEPATITIS; WEST NILE, ZIKA VIRUS; BACTERIAL INFECT.; SYPHILIS		CHAGAS		MISMATCHED CELLS	
		VULVOVAGINITIS			
HERPES SIMPLEX	PINWORMS; ASCARIASIS	TRICHOMONIASIS	CANDIDIASIS	LOCAL TRAUMA	

What About Tea?

American Indians made Chaparral tea by grinding the leaves of the creosote bush. This desert shrub grows in Mexico and the southwestern United States and has a distinctive tar-like fragrance. Native Americans made tea from the leaves of this plant to treat chicken pox, colds, diarrhea, menstrual cramps, pain, snake bites, skin disorders and rheumatism. Over the years, it has also been prescribed for an even longer list of ailments ranging from acne to dandruff, diabetes, ulcers, UTI and even cancer.

Today, Chaparral is available in capsule and tablet as well as tincture form. Chaparral contains a powerful antioxidant called NDGA (nordihydroguaiaretic acid) that has been used as a food preservative and may account for some of its medical properties. It is still used as a traditional medicine, despite known liver toxicity. Warning: it should not be taken internally (either as a tea or supplement). However, there is a place for its topical use. Mexican herbalists have long valued it for healing eczema and other kinds of skin irritation and inflammation. It often works better than many pharmaceutical products. Chaparral is sold as a lotion or salve and is usually found in health food stores.

Today many tea drinkers believe that their cup of tea is healthy and is loaded with antioxidants. They believe they are reducing their chances for cancer, which may be true, but many teas are also toxic, as they can be loaded with pesticides and artificial flavors. Investigate before indulging!

Harmful herbal teas such as Lobelia are promoted for smoking addiction. Sassafras, Penny Royal and Comfrey alkaloids may also produce liver damage.

There are, however, teas that have the potential to make you healthier. People the world over have been brewing tea for both flavor and healing purposes.

- Oolong tea activates enzymes that reduce triglycerides, a type of fat found in the blood and that can be harmful at high levels.
- Studies show that women who drink oolong tea burned a slightly larger amount of fat than those who drank only water. Oolong tea contains niacin, which helps detoxify the body, as well as antioxidants that can prevent tooth decay.
- Green tea is an excellent source of catechins, an antioxidant that can decrease the risk of cardiovascular disease by 10%.
- Black tea is one of the most highly caffeinated varieties of tea, with about 40 milligrams of caffeine per cup. Black tea also contains thearubigins and theaflavins, and both these antioxidants help lower cholesterol levels. Another plus: drinking three or more cups of black tea a day can cut the risk of stroke by 21%.

- **Lemon ginger tea** has an active ingredient called zingiber with the lemon. It contains the immune-boosting compounds pectin and limonene, which can make this an effective weapon against bacterial infections. One study showed that drinking lemon ginger tea can kill the bacteria salmonella.
- **Chamomile tea** is an ancient natural remedy with many health benefits. Research shows that its antioxidants may help stunt the growth of cancer cells and also prevent diabetes side effects such as loss of vision, nerve damage and kidney damage.
- According to the American Cancer Society, **white tea** is the ultimate "healthy" tea that can reduce further risks for breast cancer survivors.

Always recall that medical evidence will always compel better health. Use when available as a guide to safety.

Medical Devices & Innovations — from obsidian scalpels to nanoparticles

> *But these are deeds which should not pass away, And names that must not wither.*
> ~ Lord Byron

Digging though past fragmentary knowledge may further bemuse or even enlighten our current dilemmas as to medical treatments. As we are in touch with the past, we reflect on many historical medical and plant innovations that remain therapeutically useful.

Inscriptions on the pillars of ancient temples listed the conditions and names of the treated persons. Early Egyptians used stone knives, made from obsidian volcanic molten glass, that were sharper than modern steel scalpels. Rapid surgery such as ritualistic circumcision, practiced on females as well as males, relied on such crude and yet highly efficient procedures.

In 300 B.C., suturing of the abdomen was accomplished by use of large-headed ants with large mandibles. Centuries later, Turkish surgeons continued this practice using red-headed ants. Various suture techniques soon developed using sheep's gut. Knowledgeable individuals who soaked the material in iodine helped prevent infections. Newer rapid stapling instruments now improve operative recovery time. Benefits of Chinese medicine are now recognized. The plant qing hao (*Artemisia annua*), previously used for febrile conditions, is now valued for its antimalarial properties.

Chinese pharmacopoeias, while long established, have evolved into highly developed sciences. Centuries before, peas were used to counteract poisons and treatment of obstinate dysentery. Powdered Chinese olive pits used to dissolve swallowed fish bones have been reported. Excessive intake of lychee fruit, on the other hand, can lead to nose bleeds and is said to initiate the "recurrence of gonorrhea."

Andreas Vesalius was only 28 when he produced a remarkable anatomy text *De humani corporis fabrica*, only to provoke scorn and criticism from his Padua students and professors. In his second edition, he carefully omitted the perceived audacious contradictions to the Church's beliefs. While he subsequently escaped the Inquisition, he tragically died "unfriended" in a shipwreck in 1564.

Hydrotherapy, skin suction cups of moxibustion, and mineral and mud baths are all innovations that persist to this day. Medical insights in the Talmud emphasized that some animals, vulnerable to attack by rabid and vicious predatory species, should not be eaten. The rabbi/physician Maimonides transmitted his own unique perspective on medicines. His profound works, including the classic *Preservation of Youth*, challenged the authority of ancient medical beliefs.

Avicenna's 11th-century *The Canon of Medicine* was believed to be an inexhaustible encyclopedia, causing some to call him "a professional scribbler" concerning health matters.

The yellow "tear drop" resin from the mastic tree was used by shamans and Mediterranean healers, themselves often vulnerable to recurrent dysentery and cholera outbreaks. The resin is now known to have antifungal and antibiotic properties, and to be effective against *H. Pylori*.

The ancient natives carried special stones called totems, for energy, healing and empowerment. Each stone represented a different power depending on its special shape, type and color. Amulets became an "ideal" preventative for various ills. Some plant items and totems were worn to procure wealth, honors and happiness, while others were taken internally as sovereign remedies for hemorrhoids.

Red stones, ruby garnet and even Galen's 1st-century red jasper ring were the innovations. Pope Clement VII's resourceful physicians administered powdered gems lavishly, said to cost 40,000 ducats, yet to no avail. The Pope died of his intestinal ailment after the fourteenth teaspoon of that expensive physic.

A ruby elixir was also useful for flatulence and biliousness. Emeralds suspended over the abdomen were employed as a cure for dysentery.

Drinkable gold, the "great Elixir," was an acceptable treatment for jaundice since it complied with the practice of the alchemical "doctrine of signatures" that matched colors and symptoms.

Horseshoe nails dissolved in wine were used for their blood-forming action in anemias—and provided an added income for blacksmiths.

Galen is said to have authorized a mixture of oil, honey and water for his enema prescriptions. Theriac, a mixture of thirty-four ingredients, probably contributed to transporting many unhappy patients to a better world. Despite its popularity, skeptics appeared: Paracelsus, for example, opposed alchemy and questioned those theories. His astute observations were also unheeded by "those obstinate old dogs who were ashamed to recognize their folly." He burned Galen's and Avicenna's books, only to be thwarted later in his own publishing attempts.

The mandrake *(Mandragora officinarum)* is a forked potato root that was widely used as a narcotic. The earliest known surgical anesthetic, it was revered as "the Bulwark of Defense against Sickness" while, incidentally, also exerting aphrodisiac powers. Importation of this root was also said to make a man "splendid."

Bezoar stones, the high-phosphate gastric concretions of ruminants, were worn to ward off calamity and as a cure for all digestive ailments. Gastric phytobezoars, largely made of plant substances, are, like many foreign bodies, now readily extracted by modern endoscopic fiber optic forceps.

As noted earlier, the *Pharmacopoeia Londinensis of 1618* lists the use of mummy dust, human and pigeon excrement, stag penis and a unicorn's horn. At a later date, one *Materia Medica* recommended other concoctions with oil of scorpions, troches of vipers, crabs' eyes and dragon blood.

Acupuncture has been used for centuries and has become ever more popular of late. Of interest is that each of the recommended 338 puncture sites avoids the local capillaries. While many people remain skeptics, it is now known that needle insertion decreases the flow of gastric secretions and that the need for prolonged anesthesia is reduced during surgery. Refractory amebiasis and salmonellosis have seemingly responded to acupuncture as well.

Parasitic Diseases & Neglected Tropical Diseases — do not neglect the plants

"Neglected tropical diseases" (NTDs) are a group of diseases caused by different etiological agents which primarily impact the world's poorest people in both rural and urban areas. This encompasses the estimated 2.7 billion people that live on less than $2 per day (Hotez et.al. *N Engl J Med* 2007). NTDs consist of 14 diseases: ascariasis, trichuriasis, leptospirosis, hookworm infection, schistosomiasis, lymphatic filariasis, trachoma, onchocerciasis, leishmaniasis, Chagas disease, leprosy, human African trypanosomiasis, dracunculiasis and buruli ulcer.

> **Nature is the Healer of Disease**
> ~ Hippocrates

Many of these illnesses are treated by local herbals. Many pharmaceutical companies are searching for cures which they then hope to patent.

Three examples of parasitic diseases include malaria, toxoplasmosis and amebiasis. The first strikes 200 million people annually and results in the death of 600,000 people, mostly children. New vaccines can now be 40% effective in curing children. Mosquito nettings impregnated with permethrin have reduced morbidity due to malaria as well as dengue fever. Its crème-base is also an effective scabicide.

> Populations living in poverty are acutely sensitive to these diseases which result in long-term disability and death. These afflictions are primarily caused by bacteria, protozoa, cestodes and nematodes. Some of these agents, as filarial worms, leishmanial parasites and trypanosomes, are transmitted via arthropod vectors such as mosquitoes, sand flies and tsetse flies. Research focusing on these organisms and their vectors drives the development and maintenance of novel, straightforward and cost-effective disease prevention and cures. Effective prevention and treatment of these diseases could help eliminate poverty in the poorest countries in the world
>
> ~ Plaque at the School of Public Health, Yale University

Amebiasis is an infection in the colon caused by the amoeba *Entamoeba histolytica*. While fewer than 200,000 cases per year are reported, it has spread through contaminated food and/or water and usually in developing countries that have poor sanitary conditions. Toxoplasmosis is a disease that results from infection with the *Toxoplasma gondii* parasite, one of the world's most common parasites. It may cause flu-like symptoms in some exposed people, while others will never develop signs and symptoms. It is spread by animals or insects and requires a medical diagnosis.

Global Hazards for Expatriates — toxins, carcinogens and other potential treacheries

> The person who has not traveled widely thinks his or her mother is the only cook.
>
> ~ Ugandan proverb

Knowing where a patient has traveled will aid in assessing many illnesses. Some geographic areas and cultural habits (including the use of herbals) may influence exposures to toxic substances, carcinogens and other diseases.

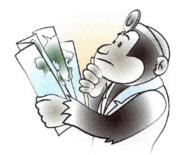

Probing Parasitic Problems

Geographic patterns of potential carcinogens

Oral cavity:	Betel quid chewing—Bas-Rhin, France; Singapore
Tongue:	Bombay and Bas-Rhin
Palate:	Reverse chutta smoking with homemade cheroots—rural India (Srikakulam)
Larynx:	Brazil, Spain, Luxembourg, USA (African-American males), Bombay, Northern Thailand
Nasopharynx:	Salted fish (n-nitroso compounds), salted duck eggs, chung choy salted root, fermented soybean paste—southern China, Malaysia, New Zealand (Polynesians), Thailand. E-B Virus, abnormal HLA profiles
Esophagus:	Burning hot beverages—Iran/Bantu tribe, Nepal, Zimbabwe, northern China/ Henan Province Toxigenic fusarium mycotoxins in moldy grain used for bracken-shoots beer—a delicacy assoc. with 2.7x increase in Japan; Costa Rica; Australian Aborigines eat bracken rhizomes; Brittany; USA in African Americans
Stomach:	Nitrosamines from dried salted fish, pickled vegetables with alkyl nitrites compounds, anisakis larvae in raw fish—Japan, Chile, Iceland, Poland
Small bowel:	Ileal tumors associated with exposure to bracken
Colon:	Low fiber diets—Upper social strata USA, Chinese in Hawaii, Denmark (rectal)
Liver:	Mycotoxins (aflatoxin from Aspergillus flavus)—sub-Saharan Africa, Mozambique, Zimbabwe, China, Lake Baikal, Malaysia, Indonesia, Philippines. HIV 1, hepatocellular CA: hepatitis B & C with associated hepatic cirrhosis: cholangiocarcinoma: clonorchiasis & opisthorchis viverrini (lymphoma of liver)
Fibrolamellar hepatoma:	to date, only USA

Gallbladder and extrahepatic bile ducts:	Israel, indigenous Americans of New Mexico (largely females)
Pancreas:	Hawaii (males), New Zealand (Maoris), USA (African-American males)
Nasal cavities and sinuses:	(Bantu), Japan, Jamaica
Pulmonary:	Smoking tobacco, radon exposure, clove cigarettes (bronchial erosions)—UK, USA (African-American males), New Zealand (Maoris), Finnish males, Cantonese non-smoking women, Australia (British migrants), Thailand
Pleural mesothelioma:	Asbestos mines and seaport exposures—Spain, Germany/Hamburg, Pakistan, Sweden
Skin:	Melanomas—Queensland, Australia, non-Maoris New Zealand, USA (whites), Scandinavia
Squamous cell cancer:	Tunisian children with xeroderma pigmentosum
Breast:	North America, Europe/especially Switzerland, Japanese migrants to USA
Cervix uteri:	Shanghai, Spanish Texans, USA African-Americans, Latin America, Brazil/Recife
Human papillomavirus corpus uteri:	Estrogen replacement, chorionepithelioma (hydatidiform mole)—USA (California whites), New Zealand (Maoris), USA (indigenous New Mexicans), Zimbabwe, Philippines, Far East
Ovary:	Scandinavia, Hawaii (Japanese migrants), Israel (European migrants)
Prostate:	USA (California African-Americans), New Zealand (Maoris), Sweden, Norway, Switzerland, Hawaiian males consume high quantities of Papaya
Testis:	Europe, Denmark, California (almost exclusively whites and Maoris)

Penis:	Uncircumcised Africans, Asians, South Americans
Bladder:	Aniline dye industrial exposure—North America; schistosoma haematobium—UK; Zimbabwe, Iraq, Egypt (squamous cell)
Upper urinary tract:	Renal (pelvis, ureters): Bulgaria, Romania, Yugoslavia, Balkan Nephropathy, Balkan nephritis-Ochratoxin A. Urothelial Carcinoma from Chinese Herbal Use (Aristolochia fangchi)
Kidney:	Iceland, Sweden
Brain and nervous system:	Israeli-born Jews, Sweden, Switzerland, Norway
Lymphomas (reticulum cell sarcoma):	Israel, San Francisco, California
Burkitt's lymphoma:	Uganda, Nigeria, So. E. Congo. Malaysia, Papua New Guinea. E.B. Virus, Schistosoma haematobia, UK. North America Aniline dye exposure
Thyroid:	Filipinos of Hawaii, Chinese, Icelandic women

Test Your Diagnostic Skills

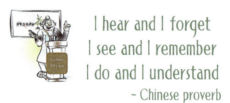

I hear and I forget
I see and I remember
I do and I understand
~ Chinese proverb

Here are a few of the patients and cases I have encountered. What would you do?

Case #1

A Yale freshman was unable to succeed in his studies because of fatigue, distraction and frustration with his recurrent abdominal discomfort. His mother decided to have him seen by her local internist, who promptly referred him to two psychiatrists. All determined that he was suffering from "maternal dependency."

His refractory symptoms thereafter compelled referral to me, the University Health Consultant in Gastroenterology. In response to our inquiries about his activities that summer, he enthusiastically related his two-month experience as an Eagle Scout living with a Pygmy tribe in Botswana. Further questioning revealed that his hammock swung over soggy soil and that his sneakers were always left distantly on drier ground.

Our diagnosis and treatment for *what parasite*[4] promptly dispelled his symptoms and saved his mother from a lifetime of guilt!

Case #2

This scholar won the highest scores in India's annual merit tests and enthusiastically came to New Haven to seek a Yale graduate degree. However, by the fall of that first year, despite the increased use of his morning herbals (curcumin and ginseng), the intractable fatigue, constant sleeping in classes and inability to concentrate made him fear that we would have to return to India "in disgrace."

When I interacted with him, and he talked about his distant city and state, it was clear that he resided within a known febrile illnesses area. This common fever belt "came with the territory." I promptly admitted him that same evening to the infirmary with specific instructions to draw his blood at midnight.

Yes, the microfilaria parasites were indeed teeming in his blood, enjoying their usual entry into the lungs when oxygen levels had changed. Treatment for *what malady*[5] led to a well-earned Ph.D. Yale degree for a worthy candidate!

The clear lesson: Not all illnesses from traveling are due to herbals!

Case #3

A cat or other feline or also raw meat may produce a lifetime of "forever a child."

I was asked to drive several hours to see a 21-year-old long-term residency patient who suffered from chronic and disabling constipation. What is his story?[6]

---

[4] hookworm!
[5] filariasis
[6] toxoplasmosis

Ruminations on Travel Medicine by an Armchair Clinician

Imagine having the opportunity to withstand the jungle hazards of the Amazon River tributaries, to have whitewater adventures without the breathlessness and abrasions, to feel no anxiety when an audacious creature penetrates the skin, or to view a mountain landscape without succumbing to semi-coma at altitudes greater than 10,000 feet.

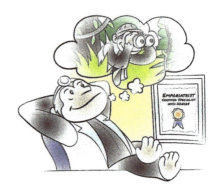

Conjure all this while sitting safely in an ergonomic chair, free of the need for prophylactic vaccine needles or the daily annoyance of ingesting huge pills, and think of the freedom of not carrying water purifiers while actually enjoying a safe Nile trip on a felucca ship into the Valley of the Kings. Imagine!

Well, as an emporiatric physician (from the Greek *emporos* or traveler), I have been privileged to travel throughout the planet, without enduring the frequent removal of shoes or suffering the circadian dysrhythmia with every time zone change. I have been vicariously enjoying the real adventures of eco-trips, viewing the rituals of the Papua New Guinea natives' dance free of grass skirt burns, and even experiencing the potential life-threatening Japanese delicacy Fugu ("dying to try it but afraid to die").

Envision the responsibility of contemplating a post-travel mysterious fever that is like the Ebola fever evident only in specific African areas. Imagine the challenge of diagnosing joint pains, unrelieved by TV's magical promise of Advil tablets, herbals, and other pain relievers, after a trip to Australia (*Ross River fever*). Just try using Wikipedia to figure out the causes of unrelenting back pain, weight loss and intermittent fever after a trip to view the outback and Alice's Red Rock (*brucellosis, of course!*). What a delight for the clinical class to diagnose the the abrupt seizure state on a patient's return flight from the tax-deductible Caribbean diving accreditation expedition *(decompression illness)*.

Sharing these true-life stories invokes memories of the consequences of eating steak tartare upon seeing the display in the Parisian restaurant: the beef tapeworm's four orifice heads matched the restaurant's proud display of four stars.

Recall the anxiety of a psychiatrist and colleague/friend, who had been a Peace Corps advisor, when he contracted bloody diarrhea after his most recent African mission to work with orphaned children. He moved on from his self-diagnosis "colon cancer" after he was shown his own microscopic motile organisms, the amoebic trophozoites: the diagnostic process disclosed that he and the parasites had apparently shared an avocado salad at his farewell banquet.

These armchair experiences invoke memories of the case of a hazardous skiing trip to Aspen, when a thirty-pound weight loss, asthenia, and a distraught family's focus on the Big C all yielded to treatment for the elusive protozoan *Giardia lamblia*—which apparently had been in the water at the high-end hotel. The patient's elated post-treatment response: "and to think I had always been careful in my tooth brushing while traveling in Mexico, Ecuador and the Balkans!"

Upon reading about these brief encounters, before you decide to cancel your cruise package to become a bedside consultant, you might helpfully recall that medical school currently costs more than three trips around the globe. Of course, you can now reserve a vicarious moon flight for similar bargain rates, but confirmation of your seating pattern is still pending.

Respectfully submitted,
Your Emporiatric Travel Advisor,

Martin E. Gordon, M.D.

A Planter's Sampler Box for the Curious

- Conserve the banana peel, as it makes a great shoe polisher and relieves both hangovers and morning sickness.
- Compulsory rose badges were worn by prostitutes as an alert to possible disease.
- To make a kilo of honey, bees must collect nectar from 2 million flowers.
- There is a static electric charge between the bee and its flowered nectar.
- Avocados are the highest-calorie fruit (167 calories/100 gm).
- Strawberries are the only fruit that displays its seed on the outside.
- Garlic has a compound 100 times more effective than two popular antibiotics in treatment of Campylobacter bacteria. Its breath odor can be abated by parsley or mint.
- An anti-malarial drug, *Artemisia abrotanum*, has also been used for the treatment of baldness.
- Herbal teas used to treat smoking addictions—including lobelia, sassafras, penny royal and comfrey—have alkaloids that can cause liver damage.
- "Vertical Gardens" look like carpets for buildings and are becoming ever more popular. Among their many benefits, they can filter pollution and provide a landing platform for many key insect species.

🌿 Elimination of office pollutants can be achieved by some large leafy plants. These include ficus, rubber, snake, and elephant ear varieties that remove impurities such as formaldehyde, benzene, and carbon monoxide.

Glossary: In a Word

commonly used or misunderstood words in plant nomenclature

Allergy: a harmful immune response to a substance—especially pollen, fur, foods or dust
Antioxidant: a compound that prevents cell oxidation
Antitussive: cough reliever
Aphrodisiac : a substance that increases sexual arousal
Astringent: causing the contraction of tissue
Bract: a leaf group on a flower stem from which flowers arise
Calyx: the external floral whorl envelope of sepals
Carminative: an antiflatulent
Cathartic: a substance that accelerates bowel evacuation
Cytotoxic: toxic to cells
Decoction: a medicinal preparation made by concentrating a plant substance through boiling
Demulcent: agent that relieves irritation of mucus membranes
Diaphoretic: sweat inducer
Emollient: an agent that softens or smooths, similar to demulcent
Expectorant: an inducer of pulmonary mucous secretions
Florescence: blooming or flowering
Floret: a small flower
Glaucous: covered with a powdery or waxy coating resembling frost that can be rubbed away
Herbaceous: of or relating to herbs
Inflorescence: flower cluster, blossoming
Infusion: a hot or cold water soaking process; internal application of fluid into a body
Liana: tropical rain forest woody vine with ground roots
Moxa (Moxabustion): an ancient method to reverse irritation using a burning herb
Mutagenesis: alteration of normal cell growth
Obovate: leaf shape with broad apex, resembling an egg

Palmate: hand-like design of leaf with lobes radiating from a central point
Panicle: loosely branched pyramid flower cluster with short, equally spaced stalks bearing flowers
Poultice: warm or hot plant material applied to the skin
Raceme: flower cluster (e.g. grapes) having a single stem from which buds grow
Rhizome: a creeping underground root bearing leaves near its tip

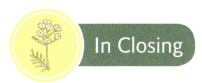

In Closing

> "The most dangerous worldview is the worldview of those who have not viewed the world."
>
> ~ Alexander von Humboldt

While to call these "final" words may sound funereal and grave, we must recall that all past innovators were confident that their stunning contributions would surely solve the world's awaited solutions. While we are aware of the foibles of people with their ongoing need for accolades and perhaps even their own medal foundry, we can only hope that the visceral warmth of our own sensory discoveries permits self-happiness in spreading some shared information.

Thus, as this penned effort to increase awareness of the past and future of the plant sciences approaches the end, the author hopes that the pages might initiate a curiosity and wonderment about nature's interactions with us and for us, and that this small book might seed a little wisdom that might result in a harvest of benefits for others.

Be well!

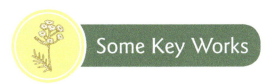

Some Key Works

Micrographia. This original 1665 masterpiece of scientific observation by Robert Hooke can now be held in the hand and savored in the form of a glistening compact disk. The cd-rom is one of a newly published series by Octavo. (*New England Journal of Medicine* 341:458, August 5, 1999. Review by Martin E. Gordon, M.D., Yale School of Medicine, New Haven, CT)

The Prudent Housewife, Or Compleat English Cook; Being a Collection of The Newest and Least Expensive Recipes in Cookery; Containing Direction For: Marketing, Roasting, Boiling, Frying, Hashing, Stewing, Broiling Baking and Fricasseeing; And New and Infallible Rules To Be Observed in Pickling, Preserving, Brewing. To Which Are Added, A Treasure of Valuable MEDICINES, For The Cure of Every Disorder. By Lydia Fisher. Twenty-Fifth Edition. 18? London: Printed and Sold by T. Sabine and Son, No. 81, Shoe Lane, Fleet Street. Price One Shilling. (Now available online.)

The Osler Symposia programs, online at www.oslersymposia.org

Daniel Chamovitz, *What A Plant Knows: A Field Guide to the Senses* (Scientific American / Farrar, Straus and Giroux; Updated & Expanded edition, 2017)

The American Gardener, the American Horticultural Society (one of the oldest national gardening organizations in the country), 1922-present

Paul Stamets, *Growing Gourmet and Medicinal Mushrooms* (Ten Speed Press, 1993)

FASEB Journal (a monthly journal related to experimental biosciences, and that promotes scientific progress and education), Federation of American Societies for Experimental Biology, 1912-present

Michael Jackson, *World Guide to Beer* (Prentice-Hall, 1977) (followed by *New World Guide to Beer* in 1988)

CRISPR History and Development for Genome Engineering, on AddGene website — https://www.addgene.org/crispr/reference/history/

Many references have been extracted from these libraries:

Cushing/Whitney, Sterling, and Beinecke libraries, Yale University
Becker Medical Library, Washington University in St. Louis
Peter Raven Library, Missouri Botanical Garden
Public Library of Science (PLOS) journals

Plant Libraries for Exploration

The Biodiversity Heritage Library (BHL) is the world's largest open access digital library for biodiversity literature and archives, and operates as a worldwide consortium of natural history, botanical, national, and other museums—and is the source for the Encyclopedia of Life project.

Botanicus is the portal to historic botanical literature from the Missouri Botanical Garden Library.

The NCCIH Clearinghouse (National Center for Complementary and Integrative Health) offers searches of federal databases of scientific and medical literature, and will respond to inquiries in English or Spanish.

Tropicos is a remarkable database from the Missouri Botanical Garden. All of the nomenclatural, bibliographic, and specimen data accumulated in MBG's electronic databases during the past 30 years are publicly available. This system has well over 1.2 million scientific names and 4 million specimen records.

The Herbarium at the Missouri Botanical Garden daily receives and identifies shipments of flora specimens from around the world. It is relied on by scientists who are actively involved in biomedical and bioengineering research while seeking disappearing specimens from Tibet, South America, China, Madagascar and elsewhere.

Test your plant classification knowledge with this crossword on the Science-Teachers.com website — http://www.science-teachers.com/plantclassification_worksheets.htm

Last Words —Acknowledgments

Credits

Editing: Jenny Price, Madelon Price
Image management: Bailey Bacher
Cartoon artist: Nicole Cooper
Electronic media consultant: Erik Becker

My gratitude to the following plant scientists, other experts, and facilities for their invaluable aid

Missouri Botanical Garden
Peter Wyse Jackson, Ph.D., President
Peter H. Raven, Ph.D., Emeritus President
Rainer W. Bussmann, Ph.D., Past Director, William L. Brown Center
Wendy Applequist, Ph.D. Associate Curator, William L. Brown Center
Jan Salick, Ph.D., Senior Curator, William L. Brown Center
Robert E. Magill, Ph.D., Emeritus Senior Curator, Science and Conservation
Doug Holland, Library Director
James C. Solomon, Ph.D., Curator of the Herbarium
Ronald Liesner, Curatorial Assistant
Richard C. Keating, Ph.D., Research Associate, Professor Emeritus @ SIU-Edwardsville
David J. Bogler, Ph.D., Assistant Curator
Chris Hartley, Coordinator of Science Education, Butterfly House
Joe Norton, Past Director, Butterfly House
Laura Chisholm, Senior Manager of Collections, Education & Facilities, Butterfly House

St. Louis Science Center
Bert Vescolani, Past President and CEO
Cindy Encarnacion, Past Senior Director of Science

Yale University School of Medicine
Robert L. Alpern, M.D., Dean, Ensign Professor of Medicine
Regina Kenny Marone, Past Director, Cushing/Whitney Medical Library
John Gallagher, Director, Cushing/Whitney Medical Library
Yung-Chi Cheng, Ph.D., Professor of Pharmacology
Edward Chu, M.D., Professor of Medicine (University of Pittsburgh) and Past Director of Yale Cancer Center
James Tsai, M.D., Past Chair, Ophthalmology (now at Icahn School of Medicine at Mount Sinai)
Michael J. Caplan, Ph.D., M.D., Chair, Cellular and Molecular Physiology
Durand Fish, Ph.D., Professor Emeritus of Epidemiology, School of Public Health
Gordon Shepherd, Ph.D., Professor of Neuroscience
Peter Crane, Ph.D., Senior Research Scientist, Past Dean, Yale School of Forestry & Environmental Studies

Donald Danforth Plant Science Center
James C. Carrington, Ph.D., President
William H. Danforth, M.D., Founding Chair of Board of Directors; Chancellor Emeritus, Washington University-St. Louis
Sam Fiorello, Chief Operating Officer, Senior Vice President for Administration & Finance
Philip Needleman, Ph.D., Vice Chair, Board of Directors; Past Interim President
Roger Beachy, Ph.D., Founding President
Richard Sayre, Director, Enterprise Rent-A-Car Institute for Renewable Fuels
Jan Jaworski, Ph.D., Past Vice President for Research
Claude Fauquet, Ph.D., Director ILTAB
Ivan Baxter, Ph.D., Principal Investigator
R. Howard Berg, Ph.D., Director, Integrated Microscopy Facility
Oliver Yu, Ph.D., Principal Investigator
Thomas Smith, Ph.D., Crystallography-Metabolic Engineering
Toni Kutchan, Ph.D., Distinguished Investigator, VP for Research
Raj Deepika Chauhan, Research Manager
Dilip Shah, Ph.D., Associate Research Member

St. Louis University
Peter Bernhardt, Ph.D., Professor of Biology
Anping Chen, Ph.D., Associate Professor, Director Division Research, Dept. Pathology, School of Medicine
Retha M. Meier, Ph.D., Professor of Educational Studies, School of Education

St. Louis Zoo
Sharon Deem, DVM, Ph.D., Director, Institute for Conservation Medicine
Edward Spevak, Ph.D., Curator of Invertebrates

Washington University-St. Louis
Ira J. Kodner, M.D., Emeritus Professor of Surgery, School of Medicine
Walter H. Lewis, Professor Emeritus of Biology, University Research Ethnobiologist
Memory P.F. Elvin-Lewis, Ph.D., Professor of Microbiology and Ethnobotany in Biomedicine
William Powderly, M.D., Director, Institute for Public Health; Prof. Medicine; Co-Dir, Div Infectious Diseases, School of Medicine
Salvatore Sutera, Ph.D. Senior Professor, School of Engineering
Guy Genin, Ph.D., Professor of Mechanical Engineering
J. William Campbell, M.D., F.A.C.P, Professor of Clinical Medicine, School of Medicine; Director, St. Luke's Medical Group

University of Illinois Urbana-Champaign
May R. Berenbaum, Ph.D., Professor and Department Head, Department of Entomology

Johns Hopkins School of Medicine
Paul Talalay, M.D., Professor of Pharmacology & Molecular Sciences

Finca Luna Nueva & Semillas Sagradas (Sacred Seed Sanctuary), Costa Rica
Tom Newmark, Co-Owner
Steven Farrell, Founder and President
Rafael Ocampo, Costa Rica Curator and Researcher
Richard Hendin, Past Director, Human Resources, Boeing Military Aircraft

CPSIA information can be obtained
at www.ICGtesting.com
Printed in the USA
BVHW020154181119
564141BV00013B/267/P